TYPE 2 DIABETES COOKBOOK FOR BEGINNERS 2024

Easy delicious recipes, including nutritional values, health benefits, meal plan and more

RACHEAL BLAKE

NOW LET'S COOK

Table of contents

Introduction:

Welcome to a journey towards healthier eating and better management of type 2 diabetes! Whether you've recently been diagnosed or you're seeking new ways to improve your dietary habits, this cookbook is designed to be your companion on the path to delicious and nutritious meals that support your health goals.

Living with type 2 diabetes can feel overwhelming at times, but it's important to remember that small changes in your diet can have a significant impact on your overall well-being. With the right knowledge and tools at your disposal, you can take control of your health and enjoy a fulfilling lifestyle.

Understanding Type 2 Diabetes

First and foremost, let's take a moment to understand what type 2 diabetes is and how it affects your body. Type 2 diabetes is a chronic condition characterized by high levels of sugar (glucose) in the blood. This occurs when your body either becomes resistant to insulin, the hormone that regulates blood sugar, or doesn't produce enough insulin to properly manage glucose levels.

Managing type 2 diabetes involves making smart choices about what you eat, how much you exercise, and how you manage stress. While it may seem daunting at first, remember that you're not alone on this journey. With the right guidance and support, you can learn to navigate the challenges of living with diabetes and make positive changes that will benefit your health for years to come.

How This Cookbook Can Help You

The book is more than just a collection of recipes—it's a comprehensive guide to making healthier choices in the kitchen and beyond.

Here's what you can expect to find within the pages of this cookbook:

1. **Simple and Delicious Recipes :** Say goodbye to bland and boring meals! We've curated a selection of mouthwatering recipes that are not only nutritious but also bursting with flavor. From hearty breakfasts to satisfying dinners and indulgent desserts, there's something for every craving and occasion.

2. **Quick and Easy Preparation :** We understand that life can get busy, which is why all of our recipes are designed to be quick and easy to prepare. With minimal ingredients and straightforward instructions, you can whip up a delicious meal in no time, even on your busiest days.

3. **Nutritional Guidance :** Each recipe in this cookbook comes with detailed nutritional information, including calorie counts, carbohydrate content, and more. This makes it easier for you to make informed choices about your meals and ensure that they fit into your overall dietary plan.

4. **Educational Resources :** In addition to recipes, we've included helpful tips and information about managing type 2 diabetes through diet and lifestyle choices. Whether you're looking for advice on meal planning, tips for grocery shopping, or strategies for dining out, you'll find everything you need to succeed on your journey to better health.

Understanding Type 2 Diabetes

Type 2 diabetes is a chronic metabolic disorder characterized by elevated levels of glucose (sugar) in the blood. Unlike type 1 diabetes, which is an autoimmune condition where the body's immune system attacks the insulin-producing cells in the pancreas, type 2 diabetes typically develops gradually over time and is often associated with lifestyle factors such as diet, exercise, and weight.

Insulin Resistance and Insulin Deficiency

One of the key factors in type 2 diabetes is insulin resistance, where the body's cells become less responsive to insulin, the hormone responsible for regulating blood sugar levels. This means that even though the pancreas may produce insulin, the body's cells are unable to effectively use it to transport glucose from the bloodstream into the cells where it's needed for energy.

As a result, glucose accumulates in the bloodstream, leading to high blood sugar levels—a condition known as hyperglycemia. Over time, this can damage blood vessels and organs throughout the body, increasing the risk of complications such as heart disease, stroke, kidney disease, nerve damage, and vision problems.

In addition to insulin resistance, many people with type 2 diabetes also experience insulin deficiency, where the pancreas gradually produces less insulin over time. This further contributes to elevated blood sugar levels and can exacerbate the symptoms of diabetes.

Risk Factors for Type 2 Diabetes

While the exact cause of type 2 diabetes is not fully understood, several risk factors have been identified that can increase the likelihood of developing the condition. These include:

1. **Obesity :** Excess body weight, particularly around the abdomen, is a significant risk factor for type 2 diabetes. Obesity increases the body's resistance to insulin and can impair glucose metabolism.

2. **Physical Inactivity :** A sedentary lifestyle and lack of regular exercise can contribute to insulin resistance and increase the risk of developing type 2 diabetes.

3. **Unhealthy Diet :** Consuming a diet high in refined carbohydrates, sugar, and unhealthy fats can contribute to weight gain, insulin resistance, and elevated blood sugar levels.

4. **Family History :** Genetics plays a role in the development of type 2 diabetes, and having a family history of the condition increases the risk of developing it yourself.

5. **Age :** The risk of type 2 diabetes increases with age, particularly after age 45. This is partly due to changes in

metabolism and hormone levels that occur as we get older.

6. **Ethnicity :** Certain ethnic groups, including African Americans, Hispanic/Latino Americans, Native Americans, Asian Americans, and Pacific Islanders, are at higher risk of developing type 2 diabetes.

Symptoms of Type 2 Diabetes

The symptoms of type 2 diabetes can vary from person to person and may develop gradually over time. Common symptoms include:

- Frequent urination
- Increased thirst
- Unexplained weight loss
- Fatigue
- Blurred vision
- Slow-healing wounds
- Tingling or numbness in the hands or feet

It's important to note that some people with type 2 diabetes may not experience any symptoms, especially in the early stages of the disease. That's why regular screening and monitoring of blood sugar levels are crucial for early detection and treatment.

Managing Type 2 Diabetes

While type 2 diabetes is a chronic condition that requires ongoing management, it is possible to lead a full and active life with the right treatment and lifestyle changes. Management strategies typically include:

1. **Healthy Eating :** Adopting a balanced diet that focuses on whole foods, fruits, vegetables, lean proteins, and whole grains can help control blood sugar levels and manage weight.

2. **Regular Exercise :** Engaging in regular physical activity, such as walking, swimming, or cycling, can improve insulin sensitivity, lower blood sugar levels, and promote overall health and well-being.

3. **Medication :** In some cases, medication may be prescribed to help lower blood sugar levels and improve insulin sensitivity. This may include oral medications or insulin injections.

4. **Monitoring Blood Sugar Levels :** Regular monitoring of blood sugar levels using a glucometer can help track changes over time and identify patterns that may require adjustments to treatment or lifestyle.

5. **Stress Management :** Stress can affect blood sugar levels, so finding healthy ways to manage stress, such as meditation, deep breathing exercises, or yoga, can be beneficial.

6. **Regular Medical Check-ups :** Routine medical check-ups and screenings are important for monitoring overall health and detecting any complications of diabetes early.

How This Cookbook Can Help You

This book is designed to support your health and well-being. Whether you're newly diagnosed with type 2 diabetes or you've been managing the condition for years, this cookbook is here to empower you with the knowledge and tools you need to make healthier choices in the kitchen and beyond.

Navigating the Challenges of Type 2 Diabetes

Living with type 2 diabetes can present a variety of challenges, from understanding dietary recommendations to managing blood sugar levels and preventing complications. With so much information available, it's easy to feel overwhelmed and unsure of where to begin. That's where this cookbook comes in. We've taken the guesswork out of meal planning and preparation, providing you with a collection of simple, flavorful recipes that are specifically tailored to meet the needs of individuals with type 2 diabetes.

Simple and Delicious Recipes

Say goodbye to bland and boring meals! One of the key features of this cookbook is its collection of simple and delicious recipes that are both nutritious and flavorful. From hearty breakfasts to satisfying dinners and indulgent desserts, each recipe has been carefully crafted to showcase the natural flavors of wholesome ingredients, without relying on excessive sugar or unhealthy fats.

Quick and Easy Preparation

We understand that life can get busy, and finding time to cook healthy meals can sometimes feel like a daunting task. That's why all of the recipes in this cookbook are designed to be quick and easy to prepare, with minimal ingredients and straightforward instructions. Whether you're cooking for yourself, your family, or guests, you can whip up a delicious meal in no time, even on your busiest days.

Nutritional Guidance

Making informed choices about your diet is an essential part of managing type 2 diabetes. That's why each recipe in this cookbook comes with detailed nutritional information, including calorie counts, carbohydrate content, and more. This makes it easier for you to track your intake, monitor your blood sugar levels, and make adjustments as needed to ensure that your meals fit into your overall dietary plan.

Educational Resources

In addition to recipes, this cookbook also provides valuable educational resources to help you better understand and manage type 2 diabetes. From tips on meal planning and grocery shopping to strategies for dining out and navigating social gatherings, you'll find everything you need to succeed on your journey to better health. We believe that knowledge is power, and by arming yourself with the right information, you can take control of your health and live your best life with diabetes.

.

Chapter 1: Quick and Easy Cooking Tips for Beginners

Chapter 1: Quick and Easy Cooking Tips for Beginners

Welcome to Chapter 1 where I'll dive into essential cooking tips and techniques to help you navigate the kitchen with confidence and ease. Whether you're a seasoned home cook or just starting out on your culinary journey, this chapter is designed to provide you with practical advice and strategies for preparing delicious and nutritious meals that support your health goals.

Essential Kitchen Tools for Effortless Cooking

Before we get started with the recipes, let's take a moment to review some essential kitchen tools that will make your cooking experience more efficient and enjoyable. From basic utensils to specialized gadgets, having the right equipment on hand can streamline the cooking process and help you achieve professional results at home.

Time-Saving Cooking Techniques

In today's fast-paced world, time is often of the essence when it comes to meal preparation. That's why I'll explore a variety of time-saving cooking techniques that allow you to whip up delicious meals in a fraction of the time it would take with traditional methods. From one-pan meals to batch cooking and meal prepping, I'll cover a range of strategies for maximizing efficiency in the kitchen without sacrificing flavor or nutrition.

Tips for Efficient Meal Planning

Meal planning is the secret weapon of successful home cooks, and in this section, I'll share our top tips and tricks for mastering this essential skill. From creating a weekly meal plan to making a shopping list and organizing your pantry, I'll walk you through the steps to ensure that you always have a delicious and nutritious meal on the table, even on your busiest days.

Essential Kitchen Tools for Effortless Cooking

A well-equipped kitchen is the foundation of successful cooking. Having the right tools on hand can make all the difference when it comes to preparing delicious and nutritious meals with ease. Whether you're a seasoned home cook or just starting out on your culinary journey, here are some essential kitchen tools that will help you navigate the kitchen with confidence and efficiency:

1. **Chef's Knife :** A high-quality chef's knife is arguably the most important tool in any kitchen. From chopping vegetables to slicing meat and mincing herbs, a sharp and versatile chef's knife can handle a wide range of tasks with precision and ease.

2. **Cutting Board :** A durable cutting board provides a stable surface for chopping, slicing, and dicing ingredients. Opt for a cutting board made of wood or plastic that is large enough to accommodate your ingredients comfortably.

3. **Mixing Bowls :** A set of mixing bowls in various sizes is essential for preparing and combining ingredients. Choose bowls made of stainless steel, glass, or plastic that are lightweight, durable, and easy to clean.

4. **Measuring Cups and Spoons :** Accurate measurements are crucial for achieving consistent results in cooking and baking. Invest in a set of measuring cups and spoons for both dry and liquid ingredients to ensure precision in your recipes.

5. **Skillet or Frying Pan :** A good-quality skillet or frying pan is a versatile tool that can be used for sautéing, frying, searing, and more. Look for a skillet made of durable materials such as stainless steel or cast iron with a non-stick surface for easy cleanup.

6. **Saucepan and Pot :** Saucepans and pots are indispensable for cooking soups, stews, sauces, and pasta. Choose pots with tight-fitting lids and sturdy handles for safe and efficient cooking on the stovetop.

7. **Baking Sheet :** Baking sheets, also known as sheet pans or cookie sheets, are essential for baking cookies, roasting vegetables, and much more. Look for a baking sheet with a rimmed edge to prevent spills and ensure even cooking.

8. **Wooden Spoon and Spatula :** Wooden spoons and spatulas are versatile tools for stirring, flipping, and scraping ingredients. Opt for utensils made of durable wood or silicone that are heat-resistant and gentle on cookware.

9. **Whisk :** A whisk is essential for blending ingredients, emulsifying sauces, and incorporating air into batters and eggs. Choose a whisk with sturdy wires and a comfortable handle for efficient mixing.

10. **Food Processor or Blender :** A food processor or blender can make quick work of chopping, pureeing, and blending ingredients. Whether you're making sauces, smoothies, or homemade dips, a food processor or blender can save you time and effort in the kitchen.

11. **Oven Thermometer :** An oven thermometer is a handy tool for ensuring that your oven is heating accurately and evenly. This can help prevent over- or undercooked dishes and ensure consistent results in your baking.

12. **Instant-Read Thermometer :** An instant-read thermometer is essential for checking the internal temperature of meat, poultry, and seafood to ensure that they are cooked to the proper doneness and safe to eat.

Time-Saving Cooking Techniques

In today's fast-paced world, finding time to prepare homemade meals can often feel like a challenge. However, with the right cooking techniques and strategies, you can streamline the cooking process and enjoy delicious, homemade dishes without spending hours in the kitchen. Whether you're a busy professional, a parent juggling multiple responsibilities, or simply looking to make the most of your time, these time-saving cooking techniques will help you get dinner on the table in no time:

1. **One-Pot and One-Pan Meals :** One-pot and one-pan meals are a lifesaver when it comes to saving time on cooking and cleanup. By cooking everything in a single pot or pan, you can minimize the number of dishes you need to wash and simplify meal preparation. From hearty stews and soups to pasta dishes and stir-fries, the possibilities are endless with one-pot and one-pan meals.

2. **Batch Cooking and Meal Prepping :** Batch cooking and meal prepping are two techniques that can save you time throughout the week by preparing large batches of food in advance. Spend a few hours on the weekend cooking up big batches of grains, proteins, and vegetables, then portion them out into individual containers for easy grab-and-go meals during the week. Not only does batch cooking and meal prepping save you time on cooking, but it also helps you make healthier choices by having nutritious meals ready to go when hunger strikes.

3. **Use a Slow Cooker or Instant Pot :** Slow cookers and Instant Pots are invaluable tools for busy cooks looking to save time on meal preparation. Simply add your ingredients to the pot, set the timer, and let the appliance do the work for you. Whether you're cooking soups, stews, roasts, or even desserts, a slow cooker or Instant Pot can help you achieve tender, flavorful results with minimal effort.

4. **Sheet Pan Dinners :** Sheet pan dinners are a quick and easy way to get a complete meal on the table with minimal fuss. Simply arrange your protein, vegetables, and seasonings on a sheet pan, then pop it in the oven to roast until everything is cooked through and caramelized. Not only are sheet pan dinners delicious, but they also require minimal prep and cleanup, making them perfect for busy weeknights.

5. **Pre-Cut and Pre-Washed Ingredients :** Take advantage of pre-cut and pre-washed ingredients to save time on meal preparation. Many grocery stores offer a variety of pre-cut fruits, vegetables, and salad greens, as well as pre-marinated proteins and pre-cooked grains. While these convenience items may cost a little more than their whole counterparts, they can save you valuable time in the kitchen, making them well worth the investment.

6. **Quick Cooking Methods :** When time is of the essence, opt for quick cooking methods such as sautéing, stir-frying, grilling, and broiling. These methods allow you to cook food quickly at high temperatures, resulting in delicious meals in a fraction of the time it would take with slower cooking methods like braising or roasting.

7. **Multitasking :** Learning to multitask in the kitchen can help you save time on meal preparation. While one dish is cooking on the stovetop or in the oven, use that time to prep ingredients for another dish, chop vegetables for a salad, or set the table. By staying organized and efficient, you can make the most of your time in the kitchen and get dinner on the table faster.

Tips for Efficient Meal Planning

Meal planning is a valuable tool for saving time, reducing stress, and making healthier choices in your diet. By taking the time to plan your meals ahead of time, you can ensure that you have nutritious and delicious meals ready to go throughout the week, even on your busiest days. Whether you're new to meal planning or looking to improve your existing routine, these tips will help you streamline the process and make the most of your time in the kitchen:

1. **Set Aside Time for Planning :** Dedicate a specific time each week to sit down and plan your meals for the upcoming week. This could be on a Sunday afternoon or whichever day works best for you. By making meal planning a regular part of your routine, you'll be more likely to stick to it and reap the benefits of having meals planned and prepared in advance.

2. **Start with a Blank Canvas :** Begin your meal planning process with a blank canvas, such as a weekly meal planner or a blank sheet of paper. This allows you to start fresh each week and tailor your meal plan to your specific needs and preferences.

3. **Take Inventory :** Before you start planning your meals, take inventory of what you already have on hand in your pantry, refrigerator, and freezer. This will help you avoid buying duplicate ingredients and ensure that you're using up items before they go bad.

4. **Plan Around Your Schedule :** Consider your schedule for the week ahead when planning your meals. Take into account any upcoming events, appointments, or activities that may affect your meal times or availability to cook. Plan simpler meals or leftovers for busy nights and save more elaborate recipes for days when you have more time to cook.

5. **Mix and Match Recipes :** Don't feel like you have to reinvent the wheel with every meal. Mix and match recipes to create variety while also using up ingredients efficiently. For example, if you're roasting vegetables for one meal, consider using the leftovers in a salad or grain bowl for another meal.

6. **Prep Ahead of Time :** Take advantage of downtime during the week to prep ingredients in advance. Wash and chop vegetables, marinate meats, and cook grains and beans ahead of time to save time on meal preparation later in the week.

7. **Embrace Theme Nights :** Theme nights can add structure and variety to your meal planning routine. Consider incorporating themes such as Meatless Monday, Taco Tuesday, or Stir-Fry Friday to simplify decision-making and make meal planning more fun and exciting.

8. **Keep it Flexible :** While meal planning is a valuable tool for staying

organized, it's important to remain flexible and adaptable. Life happens, and plans may change unexpectedly. Allow room for spontaneity and adjust your meal plan as needed based on changing circumstances or preferences.

9. **Use a Grocery List :** Once you've finalized your meal plan for the week, create a corresponding grocery list to ensure that you have all the ingredients you need on hand. Organize your list by category (e.g., produce, dairy, pantry staples) to streamline your shopping trip and minimize time spent wandering the aisles.

10. **Batch Cook and Repurpose Leftovers :** Batch cooking and repurposing leftovers are excellent strategies for saving time and reducing food waste. Cook large batches of soups, stews, and casseroles that can be enjoyed throughout the week or frozen for future meals. Get creative with leftovers by transforming them into new dishes, such as turning roasted vegetables into a frittata or using leftover chicken in a salad.

Chapter 2: Breakfasts to Start Your Day Right

Chapter 2: Breakfasts to Start Your Day Right

Welcome to Chapter 2, where I'll explore a variety of delicious and nutritious breakfast options to help you start your day on the right foot. Breakfast is often referred to as the most important meal of the day, and for good reason—it provides the fuel your body needs to kickstart your metabolism, boost energy levels, and set the tone for a healthy day ahead. In this chapter, I'll showcase a selection of breakfast recipes that are not only diabetes-friendly but also quick, easy, and satisfying. From hearty oatmeal and smoothie bowls to protein-packed egg dishes and grab-and-go options, there's something for everyone to enjoy as they embark on their journey to better health.

The Importance of a Balanced Breakfast

A balanced breakfast is essential for maintaining stable blood sugar levels, supporting overall health, and promoting weight management. In this section, I'll discuss the components of a balanced breakfast, including complex carbohydrates, protein, healthy fats, and fiber, and how they work together to provide sustained energy and keep you feeling full and satisfied until your next meal.

Tips for Quick and Easy Breakfasts

Mornings can be hectic, but that doesn't mean you have to sacrifice a nutritious breakfast. In this section, I'll share our top tips for preparing quick and easy breakfasts that you can enjoy on busy weekdays or leisurely weekends. From meal prepping and batch cooking to make-ahead options and simple swaps, these tips will help you streamline your morning routine and make breakfast a priority, no matter how busy your schedule.

Diabetes-Friendly Breakfast Recipes

In this section, I'll dive into a collection of diabetes-friendly breakfast recipes that are as delicious as they are nutritious. From classic favorites with a healthy twist to creative and innovative dishes that will awaken your taste buds, these recipes are designed to satisfy cravings, fuel your body, and keep your blood sugar levels in check. With options for every dietary preference and taste preference, you'll never run out of ideas for starting your day off right.

Peanut Butter Banana Smoothie

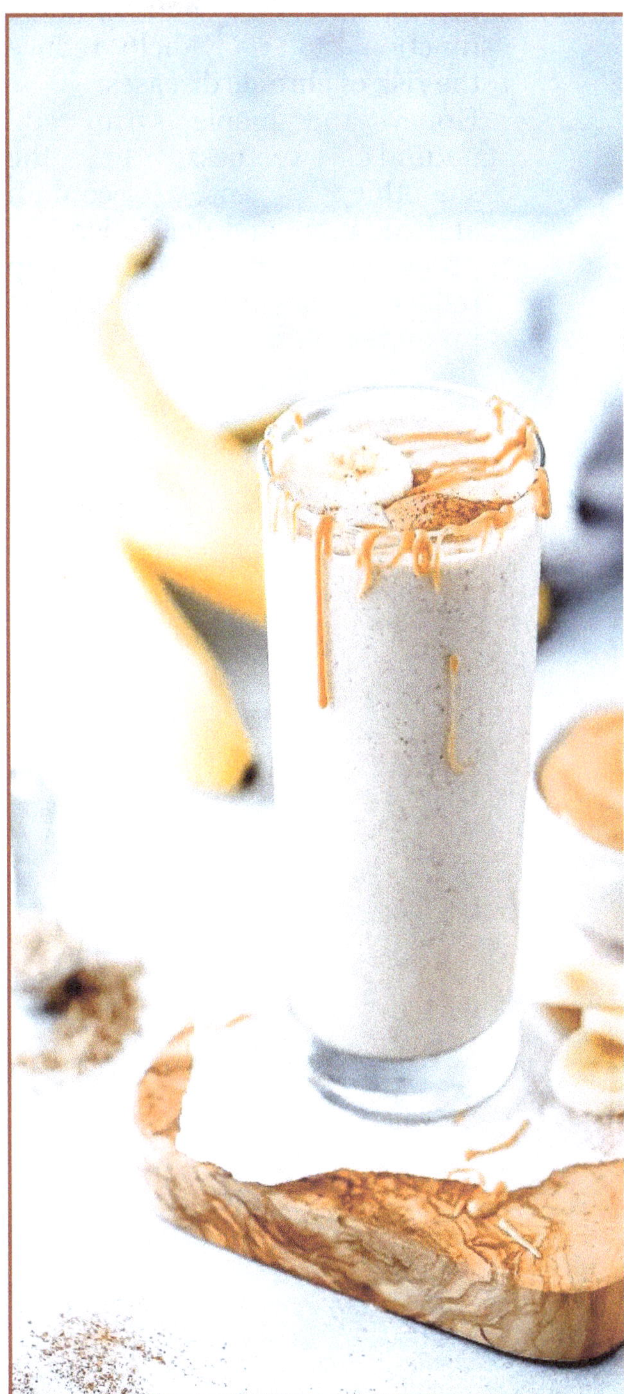

Time of Preparation: 5 minutes
Cooking Time: 0 minutes
Serving Unit: 2 servings

Ingredients:
- 2 ripe bananas, peeled and sliced
- 2 tablespoons peanut butter (smooth or crunchy)
- 1 cup unsweetened almond milk (or any milk of your choice)
- 1/2 cup plain Greek yogurt
- Optional: honey or maple syrup for sweetness, ice cubes for extra thickness

Procedures:
1. Place the sliced bananas, peanut butter, almond milk, and Greek yogurt in a blender.
2. Optional: Add honey or maple syrup for sweetness, and ice cubes for extra thickness.
3. Blend the ingredients on high speed until smooth and creamy, scraping down the sides of the blender as needed.
4. Taste the smoothie and adjust the sweetness or thickness by adding more honey or maple syrup, or more ice cubes, if desired.
5. Once the desired consistency is achieved, pour the Peanut Butter Banana Smoothie into glasses.
6. Optionally, garnish the smoothies with sliced bananas or a sprinkle of crushed peanuts for extra texture and visual appeal.
7. Serve immediately, and enjoy!

Cooking Tips:
- Use ripe bananas for natural sweetness and a smooth texture in the smoothie.
- Customize the smoothie by adding additional ingredients, such as spinach or kale for extra nutrients, cocoa powder for a

chocolatey flavor, or chia seeds for added protein and fiber.

- For a thicker smoothie, use frozen bananas instead of fresh ones, or add more ice cubes to the blender.
- Adjust the sweetness of the smoothie by adding honey, maple syrup, or a sweetener of your choice, according to your taste preferences.
- Use natural peanut butter without added sugars or oils for a healthier option, or substitute with almond butter or another nut butter if preferred.

Nutritional Values:
- Calories: Approximately 250 kcal per serving
- Protein: Approximately 10g per serving
- Carbohydrates: Approximately 30g per serving
- Fat: Approximately 10g per serving
- Fiber: Approximately 5g per serving

Health Benefits:
- Bananas are a good source of potassium, fiber, and vitamins, including vitamin C and vitamin B6, which support heart health, digestion, and energy metabolism.
- Peanut butter is rich in protein, healthy fats, vitamins, and minerals, including vitamin E, magnesium, and potassium, which support muscle growth, satiety, and energy production.
- Almond milk is low in calories and carbohydrates, and is a good source of calcium, vitamin D, and vitamin E, which support bone health, immune function, and skin health.
- Greek yogurt is high in protein and probiotics, which support gut health, digestion, and immune function, and may help reduce the risk of chronic diseases.
- Honey and maple syrup add natural sweetness to the smoothie, and contain antioxidants and antimicrobial properties, which may help reduce inflammation and support immune health.

Energizing Oatmeal Bowl

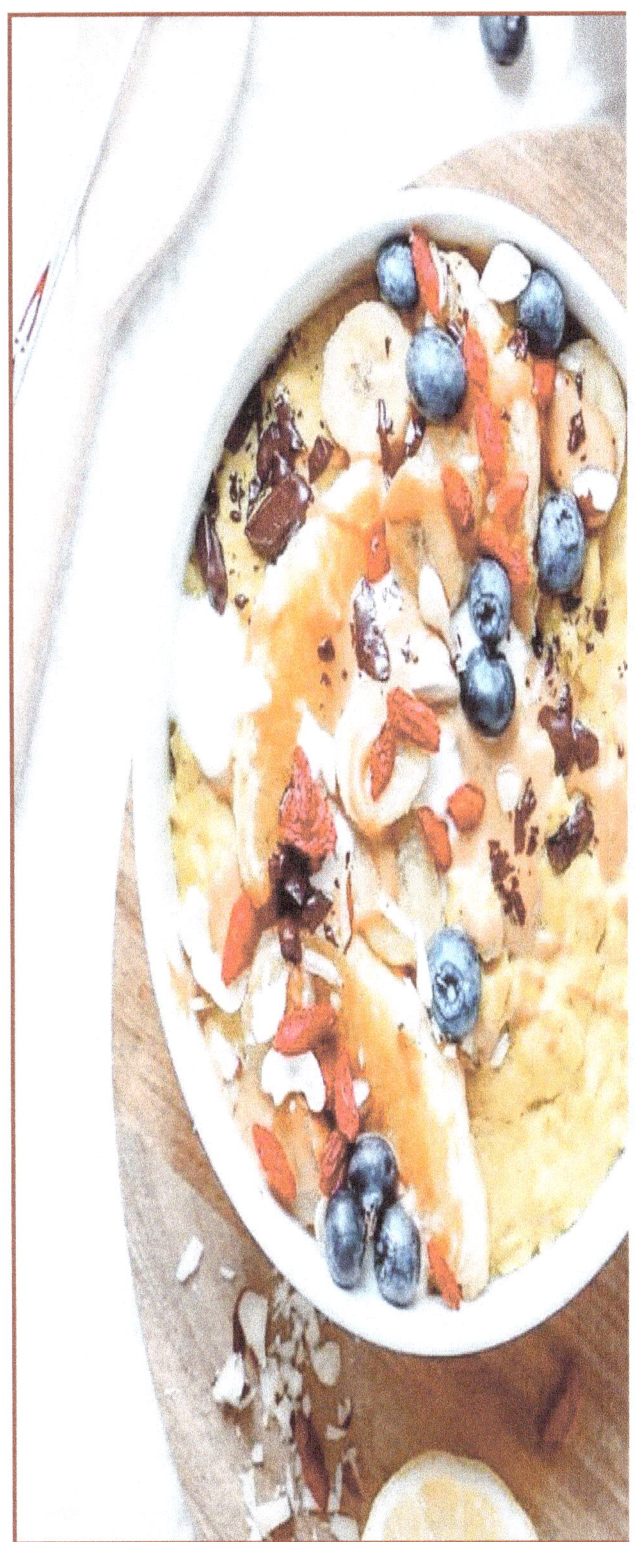

Time of Preparation: 5 minutes
Cooking Time: 5 minutes
Serving Unit: 1 bowl

Ingredients:
- 1/2 cup rolled oats
- 1 cup water
- 1/2 ripe banana, mashed
- 1 tablespoon chia seeds
- 1/2 teaspoon ground cinnamon

Procedures:
1. In a small saucepan, combine the rolled oats, water, chia seeds, and ground cinnamon.
2. Bring the mixture to a simmer over medium heat, stirring occasionally, until the oats are cooked and the mixture has thickened to your desired consistency, about 5 minutes.
3. Remove the saucepan from the heat and stir in the mashed banana until well combined.
4. Transfer the oatmeal to a serving bowl.
5. Serve immediately and enjoy!

Cooking Tips:
- Feel free to customize your oatmeal with your favorite toppings, such as sliced fruit, nuts, seeds, nut butter, or a drizzle of honey.

Nutritional Values:
- Calories: Approximately 250 kcal
- Protein: Approximately 7g
- Carbohydrates: Approximately 45g
- Fat: Approximately 5g
- Fiber: Approximately 9g

Health Benefits:

- Oats are a great source of fiber, which helps promote digestion, regulate blood sugar levels, and keep you feeling full and satisfied.
- Chia seeds are rich in omega-3 fatty acids, antioxidants, and fiber, which can help reduce inflammation, lower cholesterol levels, and support heart health.
- Bananas are packed with potassium, vitamin C, and vitamin B6, which are essential for maintaining healthy blood pressure, immune function, and energy levels.
- Cinnamon is known for its anti-inflammatory and antioxidant properties, which can help lower blood sugar levels, improve insulin sensitivity, and reduce the risk of chronic diseases.

Simple Greek Yogurt Parfait

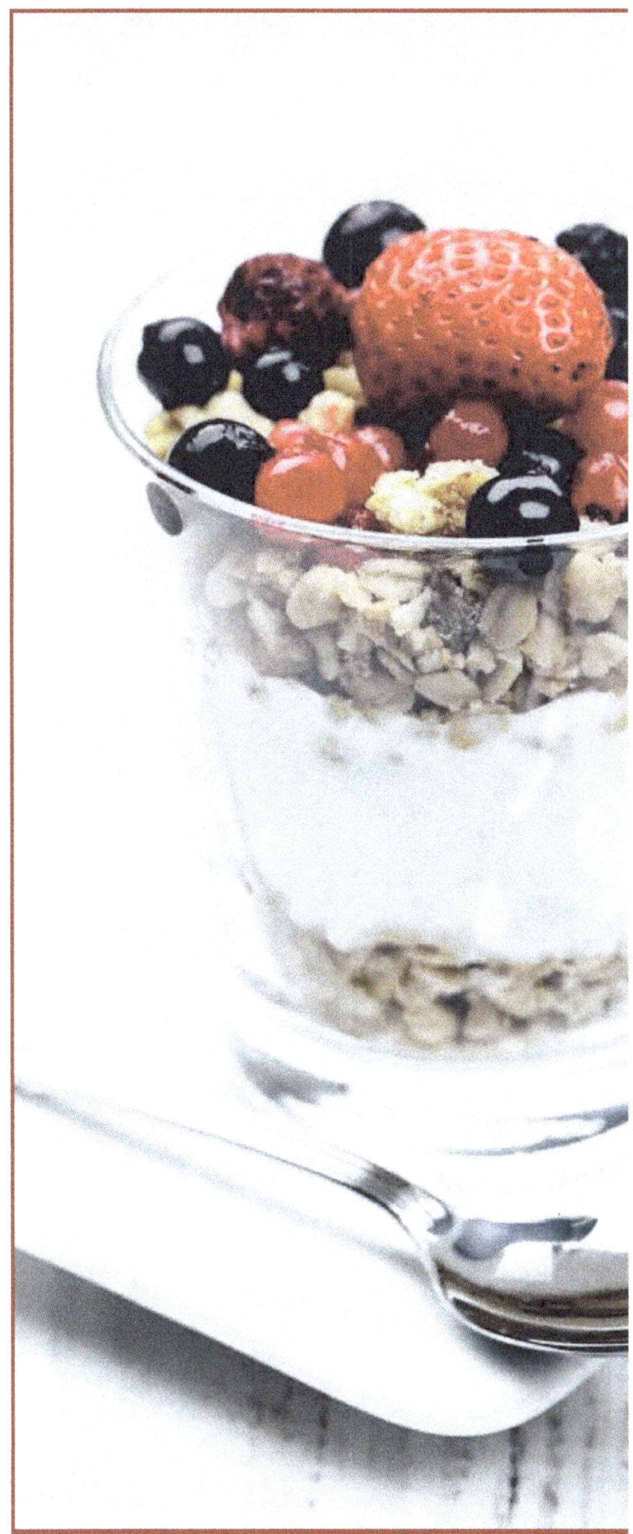

Time of Preparation: 5 minutes
Cooking Time: 0 minutes
Serving Unit: 1 parfait

Ingredients:
- 1/2 cup Greek yogurt
- 1/4 cup granola
- 1/4 cup mixed berries (such as strawberries, blueberries, raspberries)
- 1 tablespoon honey or maple syrup (optional)
- Fresh mint leaves for garnish (optional)

Procedures:
1. In a serving glass or bowl, layer half of the Greek yogurt.
2. Add half of the granola on top of the yogurt layer.
3. Add half of the mixed berries on top of the granola layer.
4. Repeat the layers with the remaining Greek yogurt, granola, and mixed berries.
5. Drizzle honey or maple syrup over the top layer if desired.
6. Garnish with fresh mint leaves for a pop of color and flavor.
7. Serve immediately and enjoy!

Cooking Tips:
- Feel free to customize your parfait with your favorite toppings, such as sliced bananas, diced mango, shredded coconut, or chopped nuts.
- For added sweetness, you can mix a little honey or maple syrup into the Greek yogurt before layering it in the parfait.
- Make sure to use a clear glass or bowl to showcase the beautiful layers of the parfait.

Nutritional Values:
- Calories: Approximately 300 kcal
- Protein: Approximately 15g
- Carbohydrates: Approximately 40g
- Fat: Approximately 8g
- Fiber: Approximately 6g

Health Benefits:
- Greek yogurt is rich in protein, which helps promote muscle growth and repair, keep you feeling full and satisfied, and regulate blood sugar levels.
- Granola provides a good source of complex carbohydrates, which provide sustained energy and help keep you feeling full and satisfied.
- Mixed berries are packed with antioxidants, vitamins, and minerals, which help boost immune function, reduce inflammation, and protect against chronic diseases.
- Honey or maple syrup adds natural sweetness to the parfait without the need for refined sugars, providing a healthier alternative for satisfying your sweet tooth.
- Fresh mint leaves not only add a refreshing flavor and aroma to the parfait but also provide additional antioxidants and vitamins to support overall health.

Speedy Egg Muffins

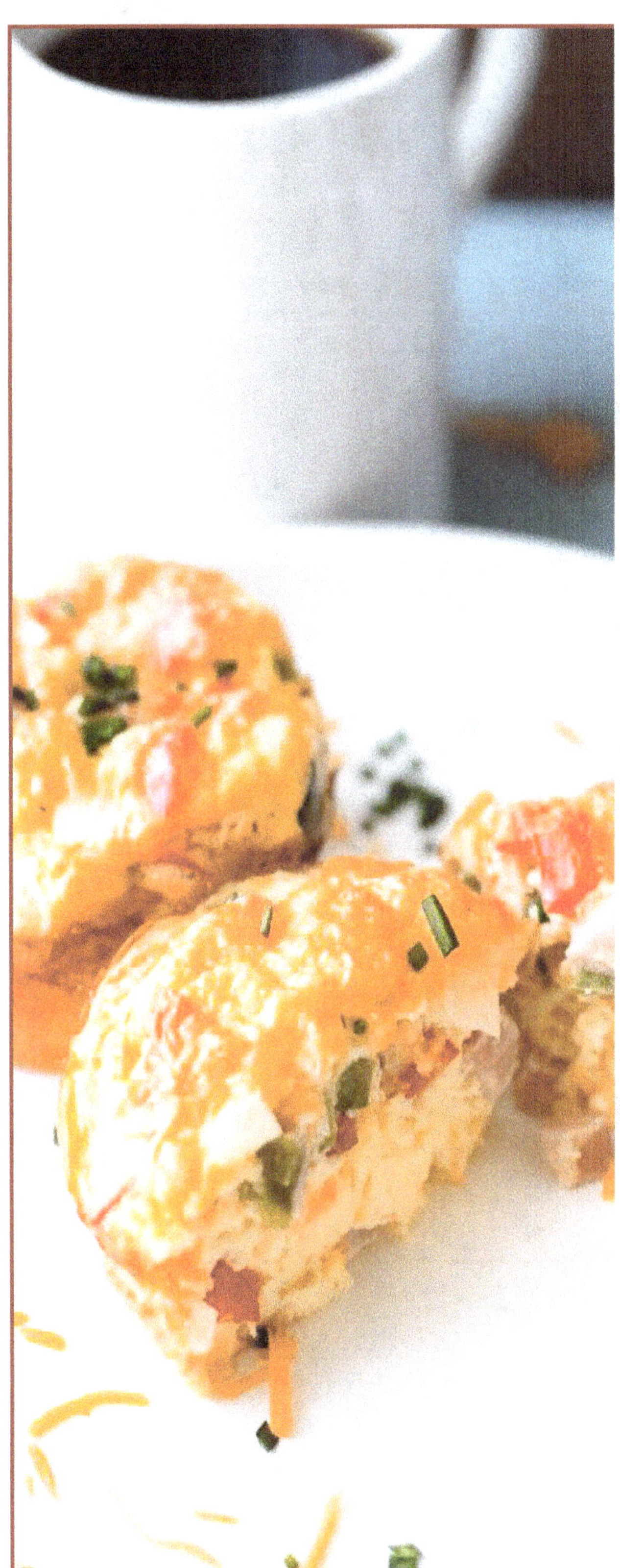

Time of Preparation: 10 minutes
Cooking Time: 20 minutes
Serving Unit: 6 muffins

Ingredients:
- 6 large eggs
- 1/2 cup diced vegetables (such as bell peppers, spinach, onions)
- 1/4 cup shredded cheese (such as cheddar, mozzarella)
- Salt and pepper to taste
- Cooking spray or olive oil for greasing muffin tin

Procedures:
1. Preheat your oven to 350°F (175°C). Grease a 6-cup muffin tin with cooking spray or olive oil.
2. In a mixing bowl, crack the eggs and whisk them until well beaten.
3. Stir in the diced vegetables and shredded cheese until evenly distributed.
4. Season the egg mixture with salt and pepper to taste.
5. Pour the egg mixture evenly into the prepared muffin tin, filling each cup about 3/4 full.
6. Bake in the preheated oven for 20 minutes, or until the egg muffins are set and lightly golden on top.
7. Remove the muffin tin from the oven and allow the egg muffins to cool for a few minutes before removing them from the tin.
8. Serve the egg muffins warm or at room temperature.

Cooking Tips:
- Feel free to customize your egg muffins with your favorite vegetables, such as diced tomatoes, mushrooms, or broccoli.
- For added flavor, you can also mix in cooked and crumbled bacon, sausage, or ham.

- Make sure not to overfill the muffin cups with the egg mixture, as they will puff up as they bake.
- To make clean-up easier, you can line the muffin tin with paper liners before greasing them with cooking spray.

Nutritional Values:
- Calories: Approximately 100 kcal per muffin
- Protein: Approximately 8g per muffin
- Carbohydrates: Approximately 2g per muffin
- Fat: Approximately 7g per muffin
- Fiber: Approximately 1g per muffin

Health Benefits:
- Eggs are a great source of high-quality protein, essential vitamins, and minerals, such as vitamin D, vitamin B12, and choline, which support overall health and wellbeing.
- Vegetables are rich in fiber, vitamins, minerals, and antioxidants, which help boost immune function, support digestion, and protect against chronic diseases.
- Cheese adds flavor and richness to the egg muffins while providing protein, calcium, and other essential nutrients for bone health and muscle function.
- These Speedy Egg Muffins are low in carbohydrates and high in protein, making them a great option for those following a low-carb or ketogenic diet.
- By preparing these egg muffins ahead of time, you can have a quick and convenient breakfast or snack option on hand for busy mornings or on-the-go eating.

Cauliflower Fried Rice

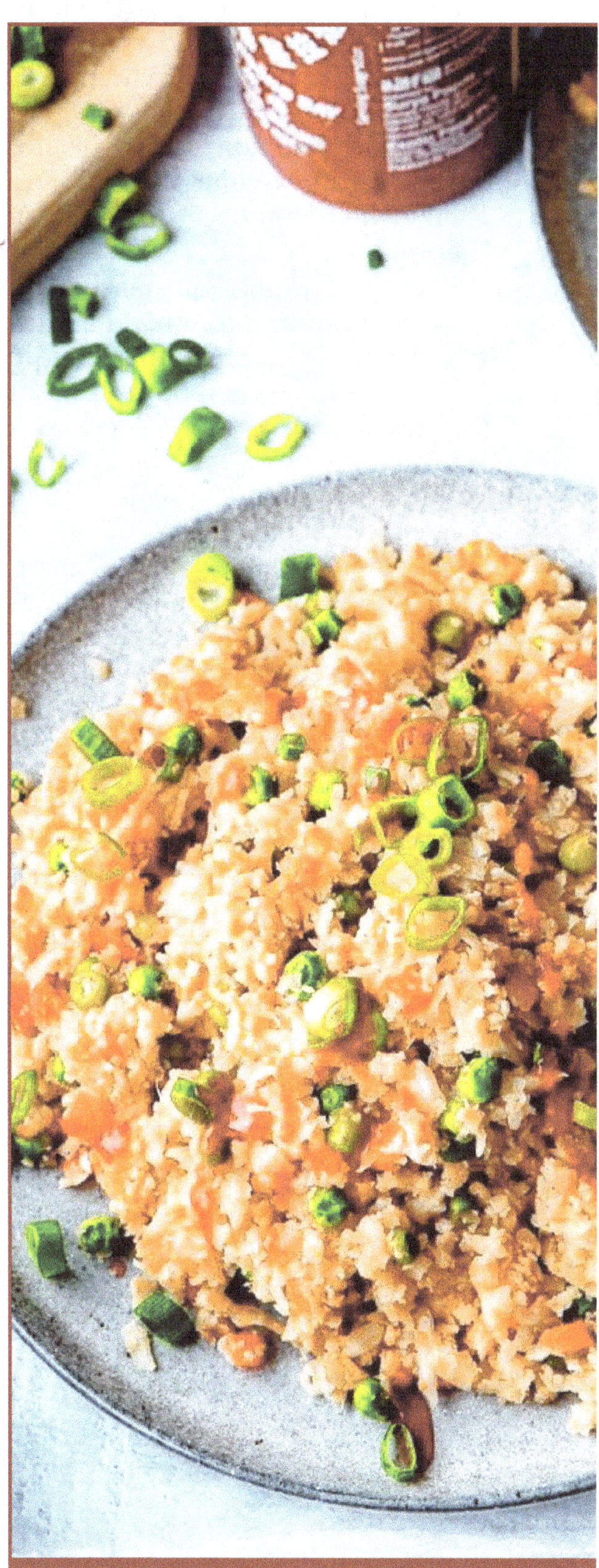

Time of Preparation: 15 minutes
Cooking Time: 10 minutes
Serving Unit: 4 servings

Ingredients:

- 1 medium head cauliflower, riced (about 4 cups)
- 2 eggs, lightly beaten
- 1 cup mixed vegetables (such as peas, carrots, and bell peppers), diced
- 2 tablespoons soy sauce (or tamari for a gluten-free option)
- 1 tablespoon sesame oil (or vegetable oil)
- Optional: sliced green onions or chopped cilantro for garnish

Procedures:

1. To rice the cauliflower, remove the core and leaves from the cauliflower head, and chop it into florets. Place the florets in a food processor and pulse until they resemble rice grains. Alternatively, you can use a box grater to grate the cauliflower into rice-like pieces.

2. Heat sesame oil in a large skillet or wok over medium heat.

3. Add the beaten eggs to the skillet and scramble them until they are cooked through. Remove the scrambled eggs from the skillet and set them aside.

4. In the same skillet, add the diced mixed vegetables and sauté for 3-4 minutes, until they are tender.

5. Add the riced cauliflower to the skillet with the vegetables and cook for 4-5 minutes, stirring occasionally, until the cauliflower is tender but not mushy.

6. Return the scrambled eggs to the skillet and add soy sauce (or tamari) to the cauliflower and vegetable mixture. Toss to coat evenly and cook for an additional 1-2 minutes to heat through.

7. Remove the skillet from the heat and transfer the Cauliflower Fried Rice to a serving dish.
8. Garnish with sliced green onions or chopped cilantro, if desired.
9. Serve immediately, and enjoy!

Cooking Tips:
- Customize the Cauliflower Fried Rice with your favorite vegetables, protein, or seasonings, such as diced chicken, shrimp, or tofu, or additional spices like ginger or garlic, for added flavor and variety.
- For a lower-carb option, you can substitute cauliflower rice for traditional rice in other fried rice recipes.
- Use pre-riced cauliflower for a quicker preparation time, or purchase frozen cauliflower rice from the store for added convenience.
- Be sure to cook the cauliflower rice until it's just tender but not mushy to maintain its texture and avoid a watery consistency.
- Serve the Cauliflower Fried Rice as a standalone meal or pair it with your favorite protein for a complete and balanced meal.

Nutritional Values:
- **Calories:** Approximately 150 kcal per serving
- **Protein:** Approximately 8g per serving
- **Carbohydrates:** Approximately 10g per serving
- **Fat:** Approximately 8g per serving
- **Fiber:** Approximately 4g per serving

Health Benefits:
- Cauliflower is a cruciferous vegetable that's low in calories and carbohydrates but high in fiber, vitamins, and minerals, including vitamin C, vitamin K, and folate, which support immune function, bone health, and cardiovascular health, and may help reduce the risk of chronic diseases.
- Eggs are a nutrient-dense food that's rich in protein, vitamins, and minerals, including vitamin B12, which supports brain function and red blood cell formation, and choline, which supports brain health and metabolism.
- Mixed vegetables add color, flavor, and texture to the dish, as well as vitamins, minerals, and antioxidants, which support overall health and well-being.
- Soy sauce (or tamari) adds umami flavor to the Cauliflower Fried Rice, but choose low-sodium options to reduce sodium intake.

Stuffed Sweet Potatoes

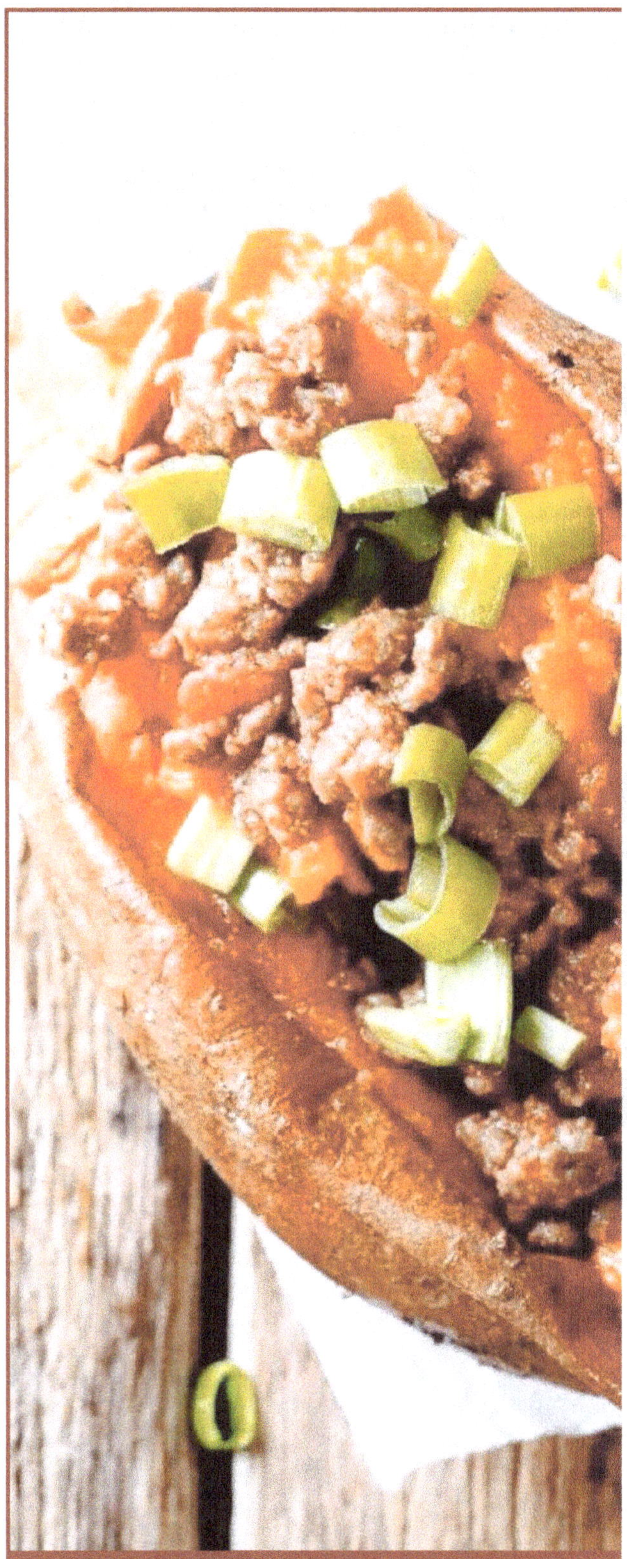

Time of Preparation: 10 minutes
Cooking Time: 20 minutes
Serving Unit: 2 servings

Ingredients:
- 2 medium sweet potatoes
- 1 can (15 ounces) black beans, drained and rinsed
- 1 cup salsa (choose your preferred level of spiciness)
- 1 avocado, diced
- Fresh cilantro leaves, for garnish
- Salt and pepper to taste

Procedures:
1. Preheat your oven to 400°F (200°C).
2. Scrub the sweet potatoes clean and pat them dry with a paper towel.
3. Use a fork to poke several holes in each sweet potato to allow steam to escape during cooking.
4. Place the sweet potatoes on a baking sheet lined with parchment paper or aluminum foil.
5. Bake the sweet potatoes in the preheated oven for 45-60 minutes, or until they are tender and easily pierced with a fork.
6. While the sweet potatoes are baking, prepare the filling. In a mixing bowl, combine the black beans and salsa. Season with salt and pepper to taste and stir until well combined.
7. Once the sweet potatoes are cooked, remove them from the oven and let them cool slightly.
8. Use a sharp knife to slice each sweet potato lengthwise down the center, without cutting all the way through.
9. Gently push the ends of each sweet potato towards the center to create an opening.

10. Spoon the black bean and salsa mixture into each sweet potato, dividing it evenly between the two.

11. Top each stuffed sweet potato with diced avocado and fresh cilantro leaves for garnish.

12. Serve the Stuffed Sweet Potatoes immediately, and enjoy!

Cooking Tips:

- Choose sweet potatoes that are similar in size and shape for even cooking.
- To save time, you can cook the sweet potatoes in the microwave. Simply prick them with a fork, place them on a microwave-safe plate, and microwave on high for 8-10 minutes, or until tender.
- Customize the filling with your favorite ingredients, such as diced bell peppers, corn kernels, diced tomatoes, or shredded cheese.
- Serve the stuffed sweet potatoes with a dollop of Greek yogurt or sour cream for added creaminess and flavor.

Nutritional Values:

- Calories: Approximately 350 kcal per serving
- Protein: Approximately 10g per serving
- Carbohydrates: Approximately 60g per serving
- Fat: Approximately 10g per serving
- Fiber: Approximately 15g per serving

Health Benefits:

- Sweet potatoes are rich in vitamins, minerals, and antioxidants, including beta-carotene, vitamin C, and potassium, which support eye health, immune function, and heart health, and may help reduce the risk of chronic diseases.
- Black beans are an excellent source of plant-based protein, fiber, and complex carbohydrates, which help promote satiety, regulate blood sugar levels, and support digestive health.
- Salsa is low in calories and fat but packed with flavor from tomatoes, onions, peppers, and spices, providing vitamins, minerals, and antioxidants that support overall health and well-being.
- Avocado is rich in heart-healthy monounsaturated fats, fiber, and potassium, which help lower cholesterol levels, promote satiety, and regulate blood pressure.

Protein-Packed Smoothie Varieties

Time of Preparation: 5 minutes
Cooking Time: 0 minutes
Serving Unit: 1 smoothie

Ingredients:

For each smoothie variety:

1. Berry Blast Smoothie:

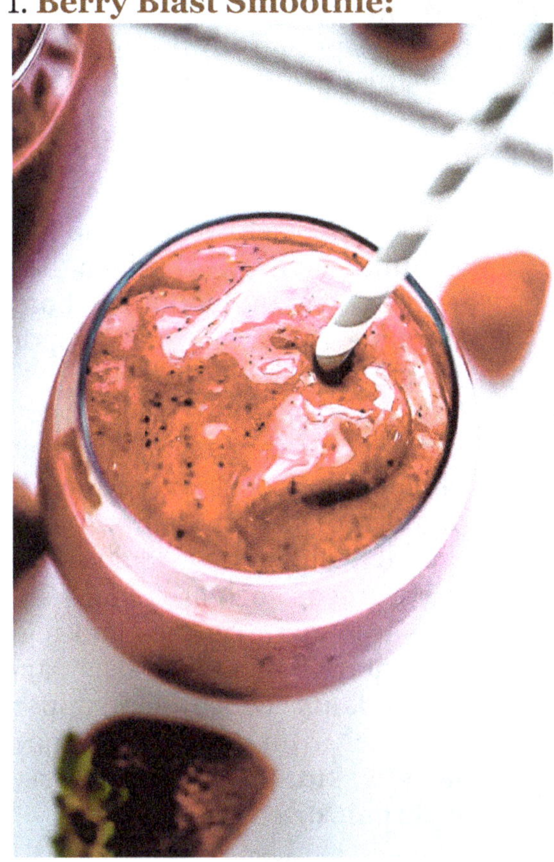

- 1/2 cup frozen mixed berries (such as strawberries, blueberries, raspberries)
- 1/2 cup Greek yogurt (plain or flavored)
- 1/2 cup almond milk (or milk of choice)
- 1 tablespoon honey or maple syrup (optional)
- 1 scoop protein powder (vanilla or berry flavored)

2. Tropical Paradise Smoothie:

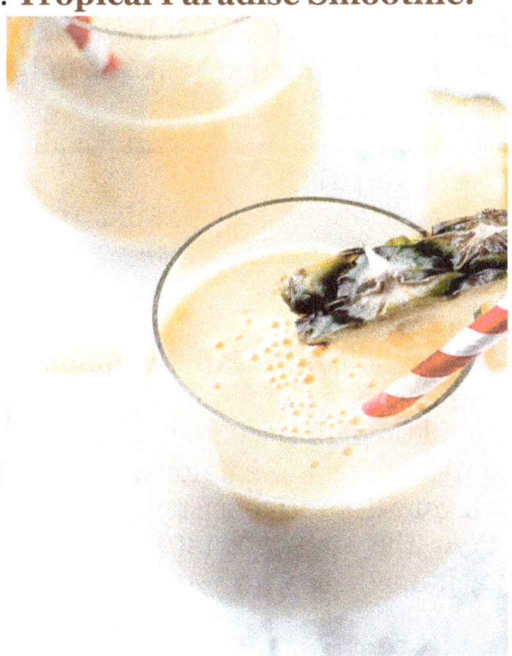

- 1/2 cup frozen tropical fruit blend (such as mango, pineapple, banana)
- 1/2 cup coconut water
- 1/2 cup Greek yogurt (plain or flavored)
- 1 tablespoon chia seeds
- 1 scoop protein powder (vanilla or tropical flavored)

3. Green Goddess Smoothie:

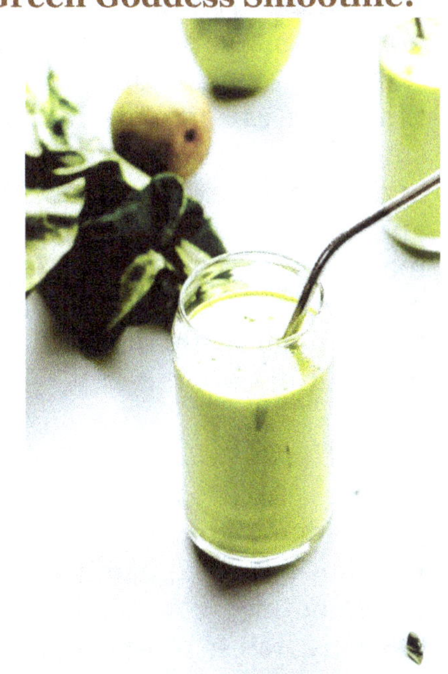

- 1/2 cup frozen spinach or kale
- 1/2 banana (fresh or frozen)
- 1/2 cup almond milk (or milk of choice)
- 1/2 cup Greek yogurt (plain or flavored)
- 1 scoop protein powder (vanilla or unflavored)

Procedures:

1. For each smoothie variety, combine all ingredients in a blender.
2. Blend on high speed until smooth and creamy, adding more liquid as needed to reach your desired consistency.
3. Pour the smoothie into a glass and enjoy immediately.

Cooking Tips:

- For a thicker smoothie, use frozen fruits instead of fresh fruits.
- Customize your smoothie by adding additional ingredients such as nut butter, seeds (such as flaxseeds or hemp seeds), or leafy greens.
- Adjust the sweetness of your smoothie by adding more or less honey or maple syrup to taste.
- To make your smoothie ahead of time, you can prepare individual smoothie packs with all the ingredients (except the liquid) and freeze them. When ready to make a smoothie, simply add the contents of the smoothie pack to the blender with the liquid and blend until smooth.

Nutritional Values:

- Calories: Approximately 250-300 kcal per smoothie
- Protein: Approximately 20-25g per smoothie
- Carbohydrates: Approximately 30-40g per smoothie
- Fat: Approximately 5-10g per smoothie
- Fiber: Approximately 5-8g per smoothie

Health Benefits:

- Greek yogurt provides a good source of protein, probiotics, and calcium, which support gut health, bone health, and muscle repair and growth.
- Protein powder adds an extra boost of protein to the smoothie, which helps keep you feeling full and satisfied, supports muscle recovery, and promotes weight management.
- Berries are rich in antioxidants, vitamins, and fiber, which help reduce inflammation, boost immune function, and support digestion.
- Tropical fruits are packed with vitamins, minerals, and enzymes, which help boost energy levels, support digestion, and promote overall health and wellbeing.
- Leafy greens such as spinach and kale are low in calories and high in vitamins, minerals, and antioxidants, which help support immune function, promote healthy skin, and reduce the risk of chronic diseases.

Sautéed Green Beans with Almonds

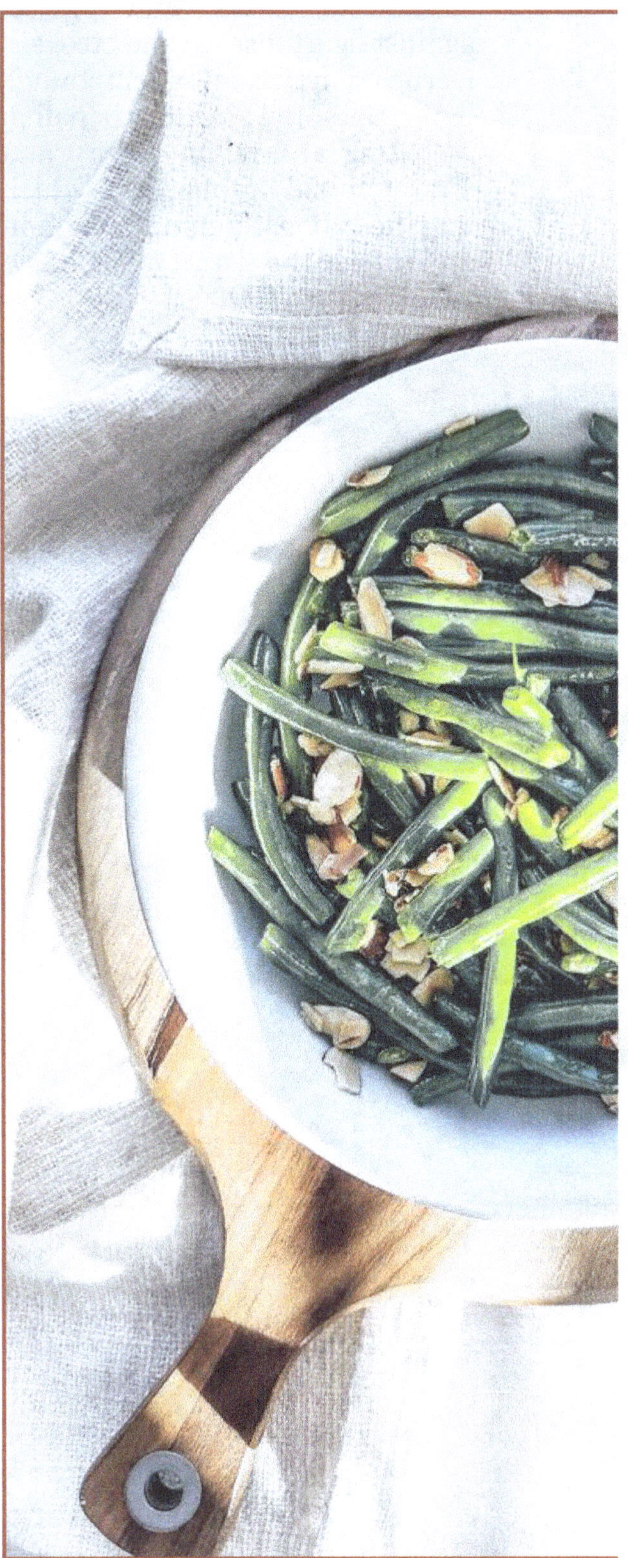

Time of Preparation: 10 minutes
Cooking Time: 10 minutes
Serving Unit: 4 servings

Ingredients:
- 1 pound fresh green beans, ends trimmed
- 1/4 cup sliced almonds
- 2 tablespoons olive oil
- 2 cloves garlic, minced
- Salt and pepper to taste

Procedures:
1. Heat olive oil in a large skillet or sauté pan over medium heat.
2. Add the minced garlic to the skillet and sauté for 1 minute, until fragrant.
3. Add the green beans to the skillet and sauté for 6-8 minutes, stirring occasionally, until they are tender but still crisp.
4. While the green beans are cooking, toast the sliced almonds in a separate dry skillet over medium heat for 2-3 minutes, until golden brown and fragrant. Be sure to watch them closely to prevent burning.
5. Once the green beans are cooked to your liking, add the toasted almonds to the skillet and toss to combine.
6. Season the sautéed green beans and almonds with salt and pepper to taste, and adjust the seasoning according to your preference.
7. Remove the skillet from the heat and transfer the Sautéed Green Beans with Almonds to a serving dish.
8. Serve immediately, and enjoy!

Cooking Tips:
- Choose fresh green beans that are bright green, firm, and free from blemishes for the best flavor and texture.
- Trim the ends of the green beans and remove any strings before

cooking to ensure they are tender and easy to eat.

- To save time, you can blanch the green beans in boiling water for 2-3 minutes before sautéing them in the skillet.
- Customize the recipe by adding additional ingredients, such as lemon zest, red pepper flakes, or Parmesan cheese, for added flavor and texture.
- Serve the sautéed green beans and almonds as a side dish for grilled chicken, fish, or steak, or enjoy them as a standalone vegetarian option.

Nutritional Values:
- Calories: Approximately 150 kcal per serving
- Protein: Approximately 5g per serving
- Carbohydrates: Approximately 10g per serving
- Fat: Approximately 12g per serving
- Fiber: Approximately 4g per serving

Health Benefits:
- Green beans are low in calories and carbohydrates but rich in vitamins, minerals, and antioxidants, including vitamin C, vitamin K, and folate, which support immune function, bone health, and cardiovascular health.
- Almonds are a nutrient-dense food that's rich in protein, fiber, healthy fats, vitamins, and minerals, including vitamin E, magnesium, and manganese, which promote heart health, brain function, and skin health, and may help reduce the risk of chronic diseases.
- Olive oil is rich in heart-healthy monounsaturated fats and antioxidants, which may help reduce inflammation, lower cholesterol levels, and protect against heart disease and stroke.
- Garlic contains sulfur compounds with potential health benefits, including anti-inflammatory and antimicrobial properties, which may help boost immune function and reduce the risk of infections.

Chapter 3: Light and Flavorful Salads

Chapter 3: Light and Flavorful Salads

Welcome to Chapter 3, where I'll explore a delightful array of light and flavorful salads that are perfect for any occasion. Salads are not only refreshing and satisfying but also versatile and easy to customize to suit your taste preferences and dietary needs. In this chapter, I'll showcase a variety of salad recipes featuring fresh vegetables, hearty grains, lean proteins, and flavorful dressings. From crisp green salads to hearty grain salads and protein-packed options, there's something for everyone to enjoy as they embark on their journey to better health. Let's dive in and discover the vibrant world of light and flavorful salads that will tantalize your taste buds and nourish your body from the inside out.

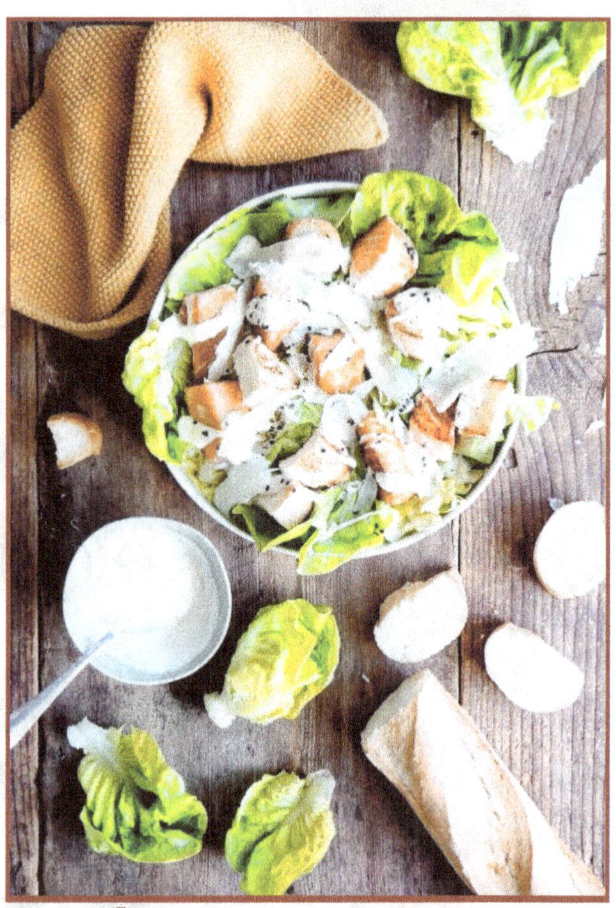

Classic Caesar Salad with a Twist

Time of Preparation: 15 minutes
Cooking Time: 0 minutes
Serving Unit: 2 servings

Ingredients:

- 2 cups chopped romaine lettuce
- 1/4 cup cherry tomatoes, halved
- 1/4 cup cooked chicken breast, sliced
- 2 tablespoons grated Parmesan cheese
- 2 tablespoons Caesar dressing (store-bought or homemade)

Procedures:

1. In a large mixing bowl, combine the chopped romaine lettuce, halved cherry tomatoes, and sliced cooked chicken breast.
2. Drizzle the Caesar dressing over the salad ingredients.
3. Toss the salad until everything is evenly coated with the dressing.
4. Divide the salad mixture evenly between two serving plates.
5. Sprinkle grated Parmesan cheese over the top of each salad.
6. Serve immediately and enjoy!

Cooking Tips:

- To save time, you can use store-bought Caesar dressing. However, if you prefer homemade dressing, you can make it by combining

mayonnaise, lemon juice, Dijon mustard, minced garlic, Worcestershire sauce, and grated Parmesan cheese.
- For added flavor and texture, you can toast croutons in a skillet with a little olive oil until golden brown and crispy, then sprinkle them over the salad before serving.
- If you're vegetarian or prefer a meatless option, you can omit the chicken breast and add extra vegetables or protein of your choice, such as grilled tofu or chickpeas.

- Parmesan cheese adds a rich, savory flavor to the salad while providing protein, calcium, and other essential nutrients for bone health and muscle function.
- Caesar dressing is typically made with ingredients such as mayonnaise, lemon juice, garlic, and Parmesan cheese, which provide flavor and texture to the salad. However, it's important to use it in moderation, as it can be high in calories and fat.

Nutritional Values:
- Calories: Approximately 200 kcal per serving
- Protein: Approximately 15g per serving
- Carbohydrates: Approximately 6g per serving
- Fat: Approximately 12g per serving
- Fiber: Approximately 3g per serving

Health Benefits:
- Romaine lettuce is a good source of vitamins A, K, and C, as well as folate and fiber, which support immune function, bone health, and digestion.
- Cherry tomatoes are rich in vitamins, minerals, and antioxidants, which help reduce inflammation, support heart health, and protect against chronic diseases.
- Chicken breast is a lean source of protein, which helps support muscle growth and repair, keep you feeling full and satisfied, and regulate blood sugar levels.

Mediterranean Chickpea Salad

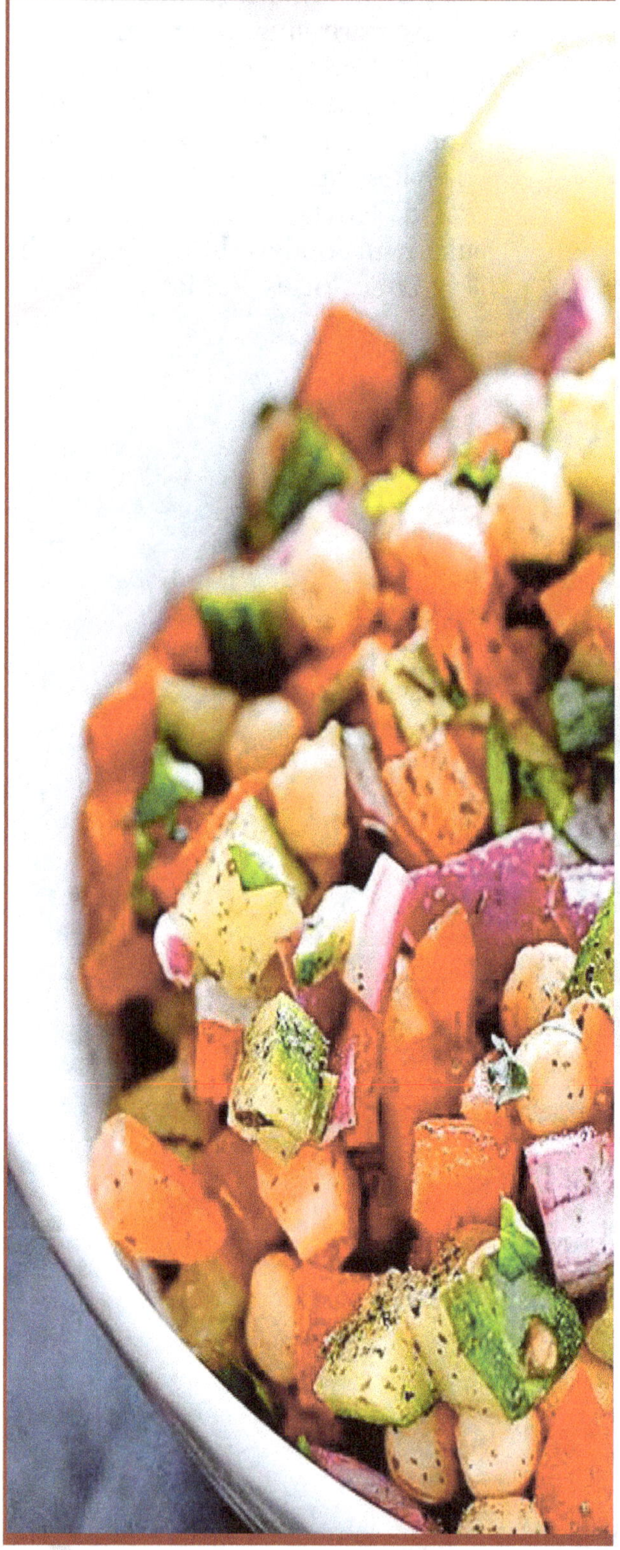

Time of Preparation: 15 minutes
Cooking Time: 0 minutes
Serving Unit: 4 servings

Ingredients:
- 2 cans (15 ounces each) chickpeas, drained and rinsed
- 1 cup cherry tomatoes, halved
- 1/2 cucumber, diced
- 1/4 cup Kalamata olives, pitted and halved
- 1/4 cup crumbled feta cheese
- Optional: chopped fresh parsley or basil for garnish

Dressing Ingredients:
- 3 tablespoons extra virgin olive oil
- 2 tablespoons lemon juice
- 1 clove garlic, minced
- Salt and pepper to taste

Procedures:
1. In a large mixing bowl, combine the chickpeas, cherry tomatoes, diced cucumber, and halved Kalamata olives.
2. In a small bowl, whisk together the extra virgin olive oil, lemon juice, minced garlic, salt, and pepper to make the dressing.
3. Pour the dressing over the chickpea mixture and toss gently to coat everything evenly.
4. Add the crumbled feta cheese to the salad and toss again gently to incorporate.
5. Taste the salad and adjust the seasoning with additional salt and pepper, if needed.
6. Transfer the Mediterranean Chickpea Salad to a serving dish and garnish with chopped fresh parsley or basil, if desired.
7. Serve immediately, and enjoy!

Cooking Tips:

- Customize the salad with your favorite Mediterranean-inspired ingredients, such as diced red onion, bell peppers, artichoke hearts, or sun-dried tomatoes, for added flavor and variety.
- Use canned chickpeas for convenience, or cook dried chickpeas according to package instructions for a homemade touch.
- Rinse the canned chickpeas thoroughly under cold water to remove excess sodium and improve their texture.
- For a creamier dressing, you can blend the olive oil, lemon juice, minced garlic, salt, and pepper in a food processor or blender until smooth before tossing it with the salad ingredients.
- Serve the Mediterranean Chickpea Salad as a standalone meal or as a side dish for grilled chicken, fish, or lamb.

Nutritional Values:

- **Calories:** Approximately 250 kcal per serving
- **Protein:** Approximately 10g per serving
- Carbohydrates: Approximately 30g per serving
- **Fat:** Approximately 10g per serving
- **Fiber:** Approximately 8g per serving

Health Benefits:

- Chickpeas are rich in plant-based protein, fiber, vitamins, and minerals, including folate, iron, and magnesium, which support digestive health, heart health, and blood sugar control, and may help reduce the risk of chronic diseases.
- Tomatoes are low in calories and high in vitamins, minerals, and antioxidants, including vitamin C, potassium, and lycopene, which support immune function, heart health, and skin health, and may help reduce the risk of cancer.
- Cucumbers are hydrating and low in calories, and contain vitamins, minerals, and antioxidants, including vitamin K, potassium, and flavonoids, which support hydration, digestion, and skin health.
- Olives are rich in heart-healthy monounsaturated fats and antioxidants, including vitamin E and polyphenols, which support heart health, inflammation reduction, and oxidative stress protection.
- Feta cheese is lower in calories and fat than many other cheeses, and is a good source of protein and calcium, which support bone health, muscle growth, and weight management.

Caprese Chicken Salad

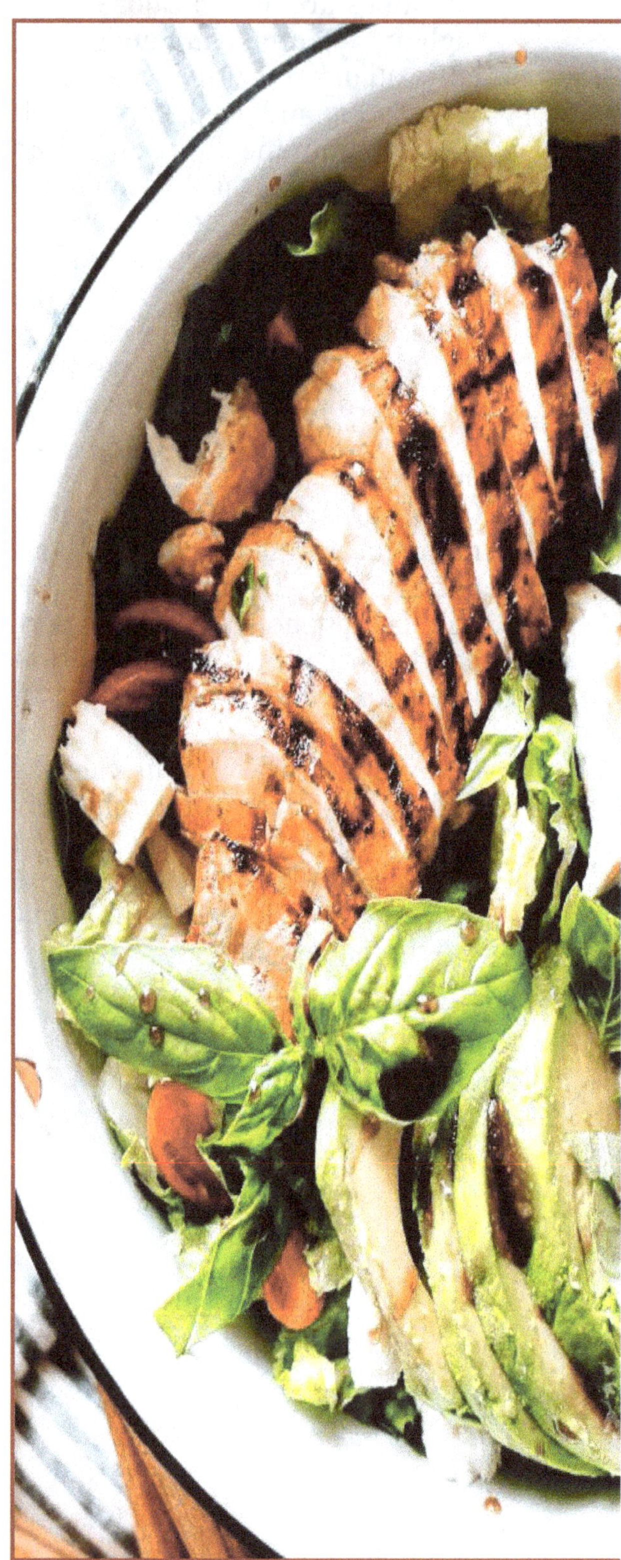

Time of Preparation: 10 minutes
Cooking Time: 15 minutes
Serving Unit: 2 servings

Ingredients:
- 2 boneless, skinless chicken breasts
- 2 large tomatoes, sliced
- 4 ounces fresh mozzarella cheese, sliced
- Fresh basil leaves, for garnish
- Balsamic glaze or reduction, for drizzling (optional)
- Salt and pepper to taste

Procedures:

1. Season the chicken breasts with salt and pepper on both sides.

2. Heat a grill pan or skillet over medium-high heat. Add the chicken breasts to the pan and cook for 6-7 minutes on each side, or until cooked through and no longer pink in the center.

3. Remove the chicken breasts from the pan and let them rest for a few minutes before slicing.

4. On a serving platter or individual plates, arrange the sliced tomatoes, fresh mozzarella cheese, and sliced chicken breasts in layers.

5. Garnish the salad with fresh basil leaves.

6. Drizzle balsamic glaze or reduction over the salad, if desired.

7. Serve the Caprese Chicken Salad immediately, and enjoy!

Cooking Tips:

- If you don't have a grill pan or skillet, you can also cook the chicken breasts on an outdoor grill or in the oven.
- Make sure to slice the tomatoes and mozzarella cheese evenly for a visually appealing presentation.

- Use fresh basil leaves for the best flavor, and tear them into smaller pieces before garnishing the salad.
- You can make your own balsamic glaze by simmering balsamic vinegar in a saucepan over low heat until it thickens, or you can purchase pre-made balsamic reduction from the store for convenience.

Nutritional Values:
- Calories: Approximately 300 kcal per serving
- Protein: Approximately 30g per serving
- Carbohydrates: Approximately 5g per serving
- Fat: Approximately 15g per serving
- Fiber: Approximately 1g per serving

Health Benefits:
- Chicken is a lean source of protein that's low in calories and saturated fat, making it a great option for weight management and muscle repair.
- Tomatoes are rich in vitamins, minerals, and antioxidants, including vitamin C, potassium, and lycopene, which have been linked to reduced inflammation, improved heart health, and protection against certain types of cancer.
- Fresh mozzarella cheese provides calcium and protein, which are essential for bone health and muscle function.
- Basil is an aromatic herb that contains antioxidants and essential oils with anti-inflammatory and antimicrobial properties, which

may help promote digestive health and reduce the risk of infections.
- Balsamic glaze or reduction adds a burst of flavor to the salad without the need for additional oil or dressing, making it a lighter and healthier option for dressing salads.

Fresh Spinach and Strawberry Salad

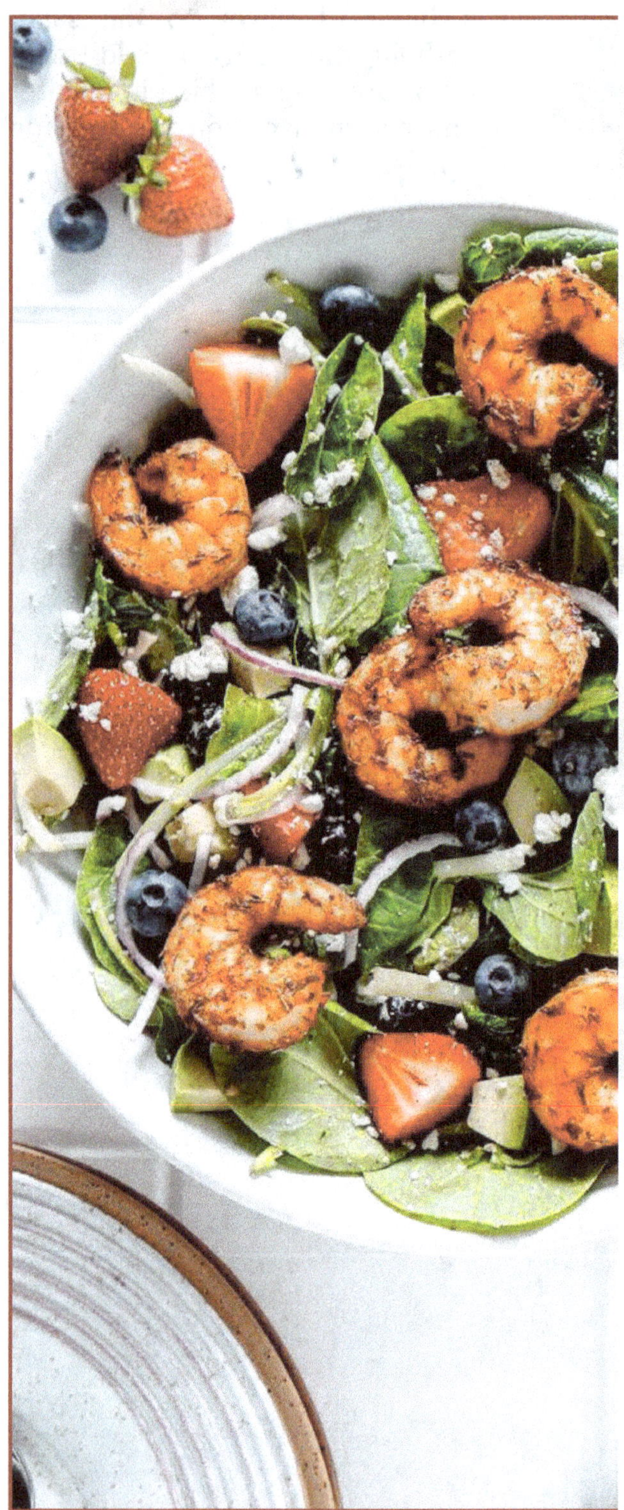

Time of Preparation: 10 minutes
Cooking Time: 0 minutes
Serving Unit: 2 servings

Ingredients:
- 4 cups fresh spinach leaves, washed and dried
- 1 cup fresh strawberries, hulled and sliced
- 1/4 cup sliced almonds
- 2 tablespoons crumbled feta cheese (optional onion to taste)
- Balsamic vinaigrette dressing (store-bought or homemade)

Procedures:
1. In a large mixing bowl, combine the fresh spinach leaves and sliced strawberries.
2. Drizzle balsamic vinaigrette dressing over the salad ingredients, starting with a small amount and adding more as needed.
3. Toss the salad until everything is evenly coated with the dressing.
4. Divide the salad mixture evenly between two serving plates.
5. Sprinkle sliced almonds and crumbled feta cheese over the top of each salad.
6. Serve immediately and enjoy!

Cooking Tips:
- For added flavor and crunch, you can toast the sliced almonds in a dry skillet over medium heat until golden brown and fragrant before adding them to the salad.
- If you prefer a sweeter flavor profile, you can use honey-roasted almonds instead of plain sliced almonds.
- Feel free to customize your salad with additional ingredients such as grilled chicken, avocado slices, red onion, or cucumber for added flavor, texture, and nutrition.

- To make a homemade balsamic vinaigrette dressing, whisk together balsamic vinegar, olive oil, Dijon mustard, honey (or maple syrup), minced garlic, salt, and pepper until well combined.

- Balsamic vinaigrette dressing adds a tangy and slightly sweet flavor to the salad while providing healthy fats and antioxidants from the olive oil and balsamic vinegar.

Nutritional Values:
- Calories: Approximately 150 kcal per serving
- Protein: Approximately 5g per serving
- Carbohydrates: Approximately 10g per serving
- Fat: Approximately 10g per serving
- Fiber: Approximately 5g per serving

Health Benefits:
- Fresh spinach is a nutrient-dense leafy green that's rich in vitamins, minerals, and antioxidants, such as vitamin K, vitamin A, folate, iron, and calcium, which support bone health, immune function, and overall wellbeing.
- Strawberries are low in calories and high in vitamins, minerals, and antioxidants, such as vitamin C, manganese, and flavonoids, which help reduce inflammation, support heart health, and protect against chronic diseases.
- Almonds are a good source of healthy fats, protein, fiber, and essential nutrients, such as vitamin E, magnesium, and antioxidants, which support brain health, heart health, and weight management.
- Feta cheese adds a tangy flavor and creamy texture to the salad while providing protein, calcium, and probiotics, which support gut health and bone health.

Tuna Salad Lettuce Wraps

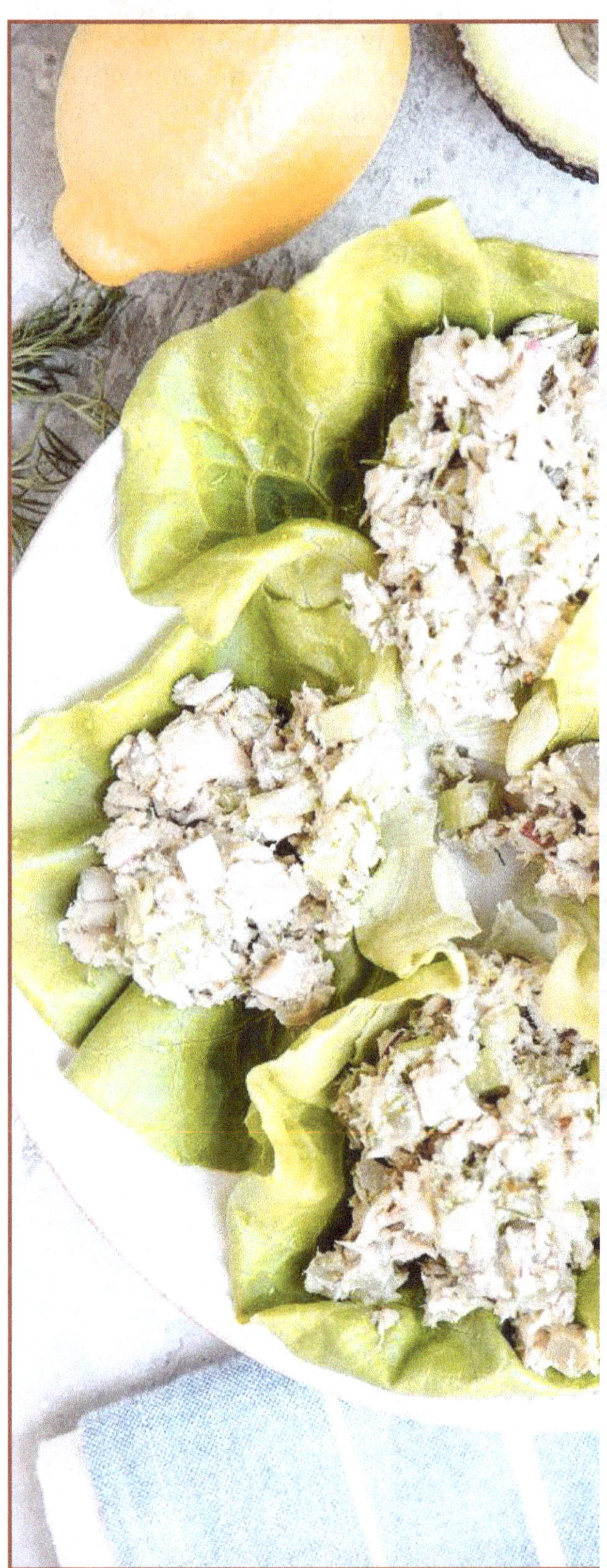

Time of Preparation: 10 minutes
Cooking Time: 0 minutes
Serving Unit: 2 servings

Ingredients:

- 1 can (5 ounces) tuna in water, drained
- 1/4 cup mayonnaise (or Greek yogurt for a lighter option)
- 1 tablespoon Dijon mustard
- 1/4 cup diced celery
- 4 large lettuce leaves (such as romaine or iceberg)
- Salt and pepper to taste

Procedures:

1. In a mixing bowl, combine the drained tuna, mayonnaise (or Greek yogurt), Dijon mustard, and diced celery. Stir until well combined.
2. Season the tuna salad mixture with salt and pepper to taste. Adjust the seasoning according to your preference.
3. Lay out the lettuce leaves on a flat surface.
4. Spoon the tuna salad mixture onto the center of each lettuce leaf, dividing it evenly between the four leaves.
5. Gently roll up each lettuce leaf around the tuna salad filling to form a wrap.
6. Secure the wraps with toothpicks if necessary.
7. Serve the Tuna Salad Lettuce Wraps immediately, and enjoy!

Cooking Tips:

- Choose lettuce leaves that are large and sturdy enough to hold the tuna salad filling without tearing.
- Feel free to customize the tuna salad filling with additional ingredients, such as diced onions, bell peppers, pickles, or hard-boiled eggs, for added flavor and texture.

- For a spicier kick, you can add a dash of hot sauce or chopped jalapeños to the tuna salad mixture.
- Serve the lettuce wraps with a side of sliced vegetables, such as carrots, cucumbers, or cherry tomatoes, for added crunch and nutrition.

Nutritional Values:
- Calories: Approximately 200 kcal per serving (2 wraps)
- Protein: Approximately 15g per serving
- Carbohydrates: Approximately 5g per serving
- Fat: Approximately 15g per serving
- Fiber: Approximately 1g per serving

Health Benefits:
- Tuna is a lean source of protein that's low in calories and saturated fat, but high in omega-3 fatty acids, which support heart health, brain function, and inflammation reduction.
- Mayonnaise provides creaminess and flavor to the tuna salad, but you can use Greek yogurt as a lighter and lower-fat alternative that's still rich in protein and probiotics.
- Dijon mustard adds tanginess and depth of flavor to the tuna salad without the need for additional ingredients or seasonings.
- Celery adds crunch and freshness to the tuna salad, as well as vitamins, minerals, and antioxidants that support digestion, hydration, and immune function.
- Lettuce leaves are low in calories and carbohydrates but rich in vitamins, minerals, and antioxidants, including vitamin A, vitamin K, and folate, which promote eye health, bone health, and overall well-being.

Tangy Cucumber and Tomato Salad

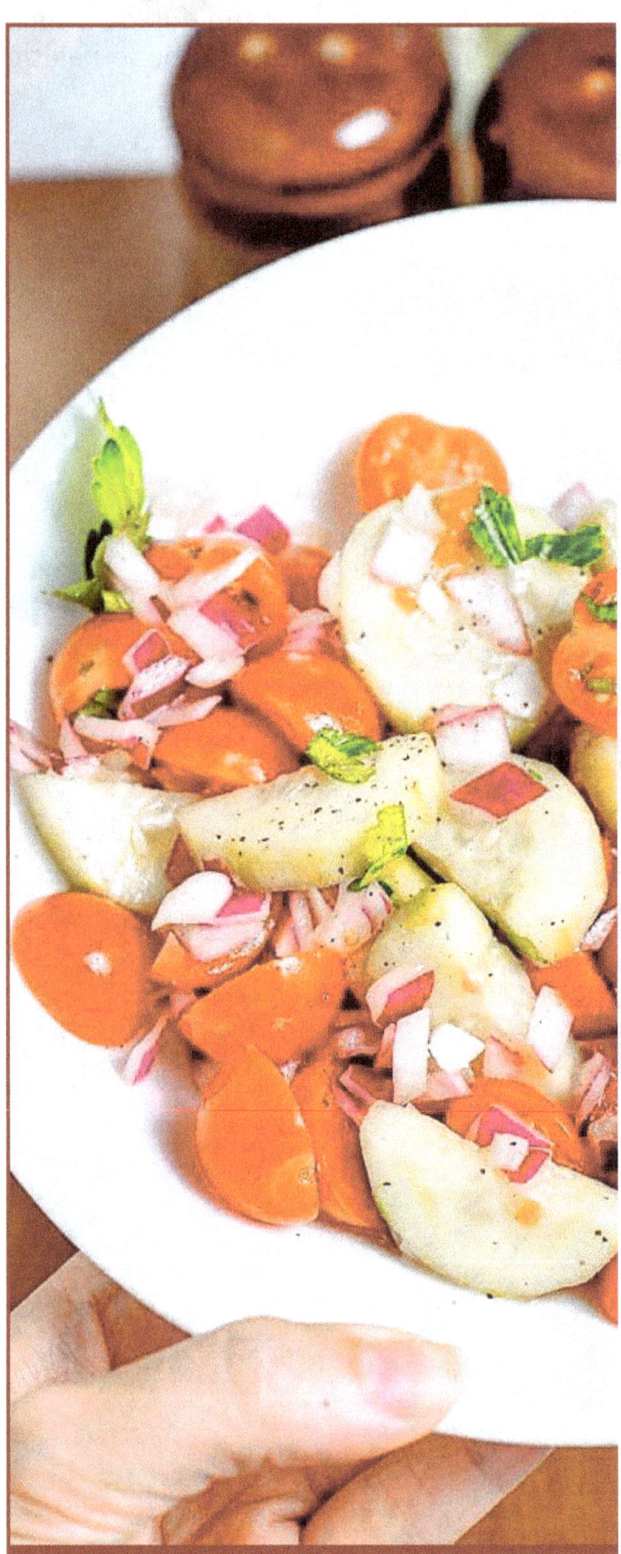

Time of Preparation: 10 minutes
Cooking Time: 0 minutes
Serving Unit: 2 servings

Ingredients:
- 1 large cucumber, thinly sliced
- 2 ripe tomatoes, diced
- 1/4 red onion, thinly sliced
- 2 tablespoons fresh lemon juice
- Salt and pepper to taste

Procedures:
1. In a large mixing bowl, combine the thinly sliced cucumber, diced tomatoes, and thinly sliced red onion.
2. Drizzle fresh lemon juice over the salad ingredients.
3. Season the salad with salt and pepper to taste.
4. Toss the salad until everything is evenly coated with the lemon juice.
5. Divide the salad mixture evenly between two serving plates.
6. Serve immediately and enjoy!

Cooking Tips:
- For added flavor, you can sprinkle fresh herbs such as parsley or mint leaves over the salad before serving.
- Feel free to customize your salad with additional ingredients such as diced bell peppers or olives if desired.
- To make the salad ahead of time, you can prepare the dressing and chop the vegetables in advance, then assemble the salad just before serving to prevent the vegetables from becoming soggy.

Nutritional Values:
- Calories: Approximately 40 kcal per serving
- Protein: Approximately 1g per serving

- Carbohydrates: Approximately 10g per serving
- Fat: Approximately 0g per serving
- Fiber: Approximately 2g per serving

Health Benefits:
- Cucumbers are low in calories and high in water content, making them hydrating and refreshing. They also contain vitamins, minerals, and antioxidants, such as vitamin K, potassium, and flavonoids, which help reduce inflammation, support hydration, and promote healthy skin.
- Tomatoes are rich in vitamins, minerals, and antioxidants, such as vitamin C, potassium, and lycopene, which help boost immune function, support heart health, and protect against certain types of cancer.
- Red onions add a tangy flavor and crunchy texture to the salad while providing vitamins, minerals, and antioxidants, such as vitamin C, manganese, and quercetin, which help support immune function, regulate blood sugar levels, and reduce inflammation.
- Lemon juice adds a tangy flavor to the salad while providing vitamin C and antioxidants, which help boost immune function, support digestion, and detoxify the body.

Protein-Packed Chicken Salad

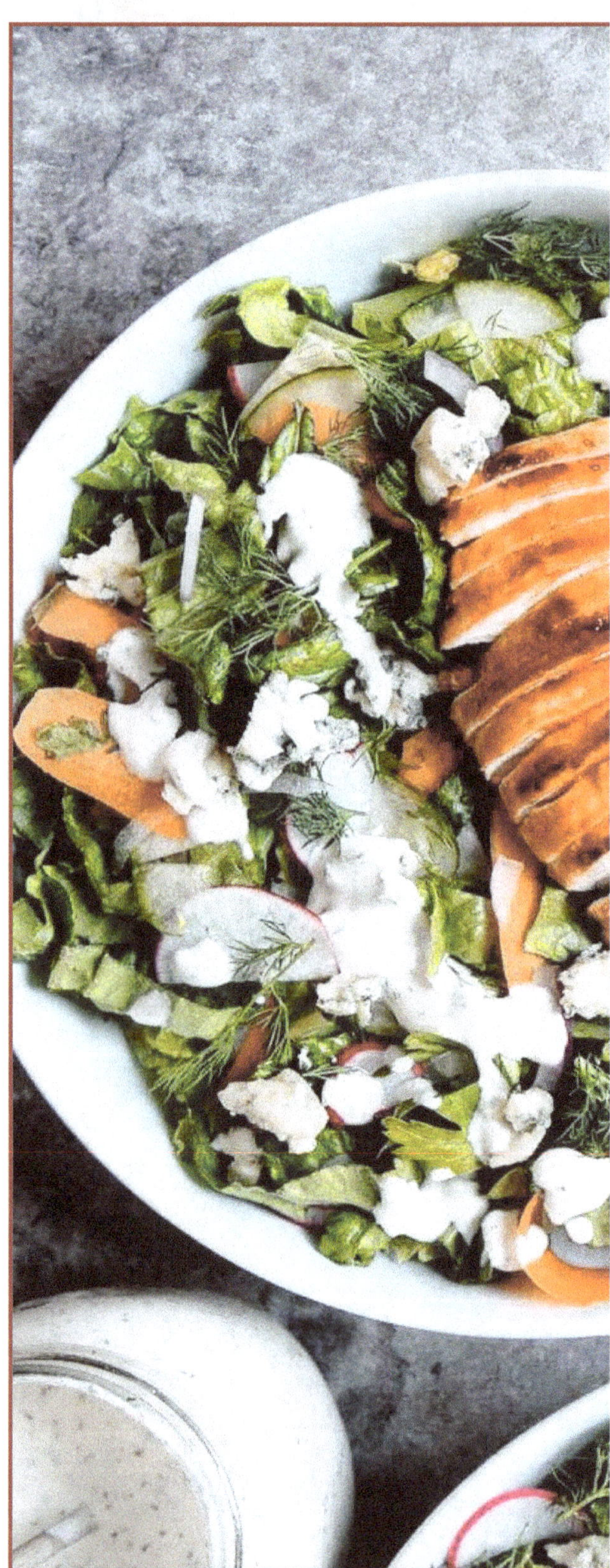

Time of Preparation: 15 minutes
Cooking Time: 15 minutes
Serving Unit: 2 servings

Ingredients:
- 2 boneless, skinless chicken breasts
- 4 cups mixed salad greens
- 1/2 cup cherry tomatoes, halved
- 1/4 cup sliced almonds
- 2 tablespoons balsamic vinaigrette dressing (store-bought or homemade)

Procedures:
1. Season the chicken breasts with salt and pepper on both sides.
2. Heat a grill pan or skillet over medium-high heat. Cook the chicken breasts for 6-7 minutes on each side, or until cooked through and no longer pink in the center. Remove from heat and let them rest for a few minutes.
3. Meanwhile, in a large mixing bowl, combine the mixed salad greens and cherry tomatoes.
4. Slice the cooked chicken breasts into strips or cubes and add them to the bowl with the salad greens and tomatoes.
5. Drizzle balsamic vinaigrette dressing over the salad mixture.
6. Toss the salad until everything is evenly coated with the dressing.
7. Divide the salad mixture evenly between two serving plates.
8. Sprinkle sliced almonds over the top of each salad.
9. Serve immediately and enjoy!

Cooking Tips:
- For added flavor, you can marinate the chicken breasts in a mixture of olive oil, lemon juice, garlic, and herbs for 30 minutes before grilling.
- Make sure to let the chicken breasts rest for a few minutes

after cooking to allow the juices to redistribute, resulting in juicier and more flavorful chicken.
- Feel free to customize your salad with additional ingredients such as avocado slices, cucumber, red onion, or crumbled feta cheese for added flavor, texture, and nutrition.
- To save time, you can use pre-cooked or rotisserie chicken instead of grilling your own chicken breasts.

Nutritional Values:
- Calories: Approximately 300 kcal per serving
- Protein: Approximately 30g per serving
- Carbohydrates: Approximately 12g per serving
- Fat: Approximately 15g per serving
- Fiber: Approximately 5g per serving

Health Benefits:
- Chicken is a lean source of protein that's rich in essential nutrients such as vitamins B6 and B12, niacin, phosphorus, and selenium, which support muscle growth and repair, immune function, and overall health.
- Mixed salad greens provide a variety of vitamins, minerals, and antioxidants, such as vitamins A, C, and K, folate, iron, and phytonutrients, which help reduce inflammation, support digestion, and protect against chronic diseases.
- Cherry tomatoes are rich in vitamins, minerals, and antioxidants, such as vitamin C, potassium, and lycopene, which help boost immune function, support heart health, and protect against certain types of cancer.
- Almonds are a good source of healthy fats, protein, fiber, and essential nutrients, such as vitamin E, magnesium, and antioxidants, which support brain health, heart health, and weight management.
- Balsamic vinaigrette dressing adds a tangy flavor to the salad while providing healthy fats and antioxidants from the olive oil and balsamic vinegar.

Garlic Butter Shrimp Pasta

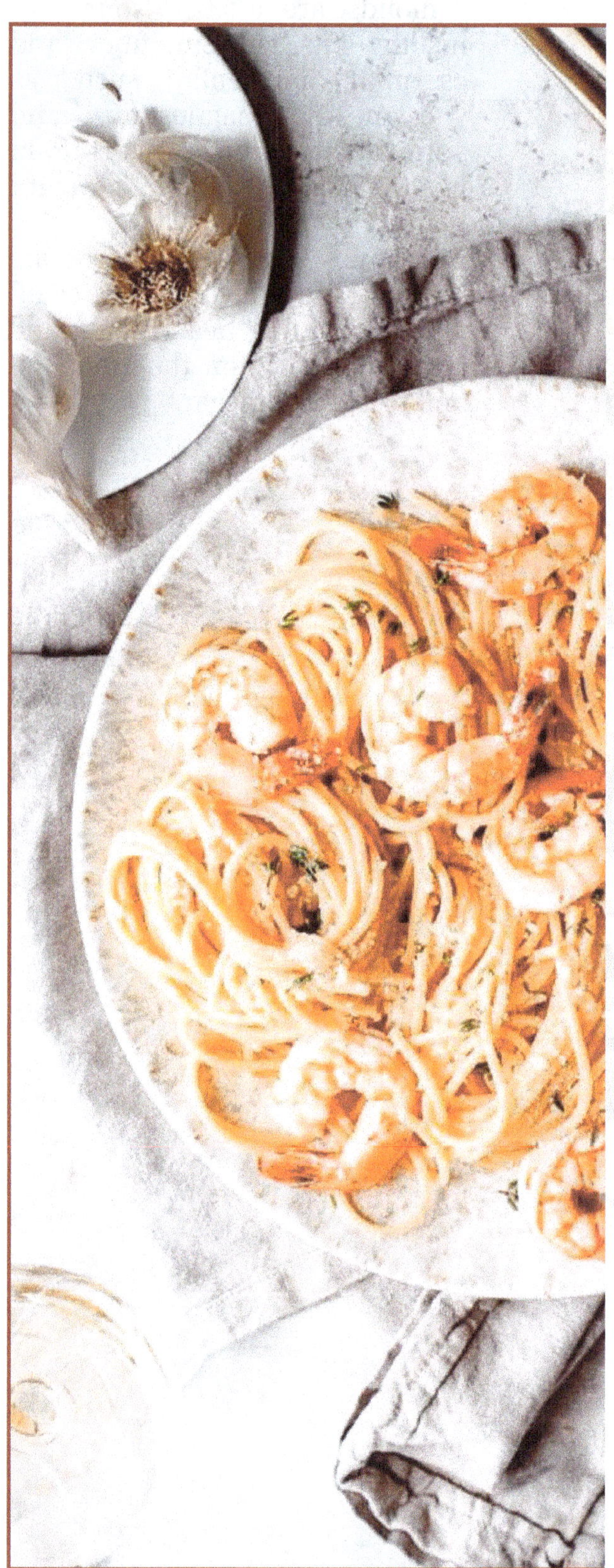

Time of Preparation: 10 minutes
Cooking Time: 15 minutes
Serving Unit: 2 servings

Ingredients:
- 8 ounces linguine pasta
- 8 ounces large shrimp, peeled and deveined
- 4 cloves garlic, minced
- 2 tablespoons unsalted butter
- 1/4 teaspoon red pepper flakes (optional)
- Salt and pepper to taste
- Fresh parsley, chopped, for garnish (optional)
- Grated Parmesan cheese, for serving (optional)

Procedures:
1. Cook the linguine pasta according to the package instructions until al dente. Drain and set aside.
2. In a large skillet, melt the butter over medium heat. Add the minced garlic and red pepper flakes (if using) to the skillet and sauté for 1-2 minutes, until fragrant.
3. Add the shrimp to the skillet and season with salt and pepper. Cook for 2-3 minutes on each side, until the shrimp are pink and opaque.
4. Add the cooked pasta to the skillet with the shrimp and garlic butter sauce. Toss everything together until the pasta is well coated in the sauce and heated through.
5. Remove the skillet from the heat and garnish with chopped parsley and grated Parmesan cheese, if desired.
6. Serve the Garlic Butter Shrimp Pasta immediately, and enjoy!

Cooking Tips:
- For added flavor, you can use a combination of olive oil and butter to sauté the garlic.

- Make sure not to overcook the shrimp, as they can become tough and rubbery. Cook them just until they turn pink and opaque.
- Feel free to customize the recipe with your favorite pasta shape or additional ingredients, such as cherry tomatoes, spinach, or mushrooms.
- Serve the pasta with a side salad or crusty bread for a complete meal.

Nutritional Values:
- Calories: Approximately 400 kcal per serving
- Protein: Approximately 20g per serving
- Carbohydrates: Approximately 40g per serving
- Fat: Approximately 15g per serving
- Fiber: Approximately 2g per serving

Health Benefits:
- Shrimp is a lean source of protein that's low in calories and saturated fat, making it a heart-healthy choice for protein.
- Garlic is known for its immune-boosting properties and may help lower cholesterol levels and blood pressure.
- Butter adds richness and flavor to the dish, but you can use a smaller amount or substitute with olive oil for a lighter option.
- Red pepper flakes add a hint of spice and may help boost metabolism and aid in digestion.
- Parsley is a good source of vitamin K, vitamin C, and antioxidants, which promote bone health and support immune function.

Chapter 4: Satisfying One-Pan Meals

Chapter 4: Satisfying One-Pan Meals

Welcome to Chapter 4, where we delve into the world of satisfying one-pan meals. In this chapter, I'll explore recipes that are not only quick and easy to prepare but also minimize cleanup by utilizing just one pan for cooking. These meals are perfect for busy weeknights when you want a delicious and nutritious meal without spending hours in the kitchen or dealing with a sink full of dishes afterward.

From hearty skillet dinners to flavorful sheet pan suppers, these recipes are designed to streamline your cooking process while still delivering on taste and nutrition. Whether you're craving comforting classics or adventurous flavors, you'll find plenty of inspiration in this chapter to satisfy your hunger and simplify your mealtime routine. Let's dive in and discover the joy of one-pan cooking!

Lemon Herb Chicken with Roasted Vegetables

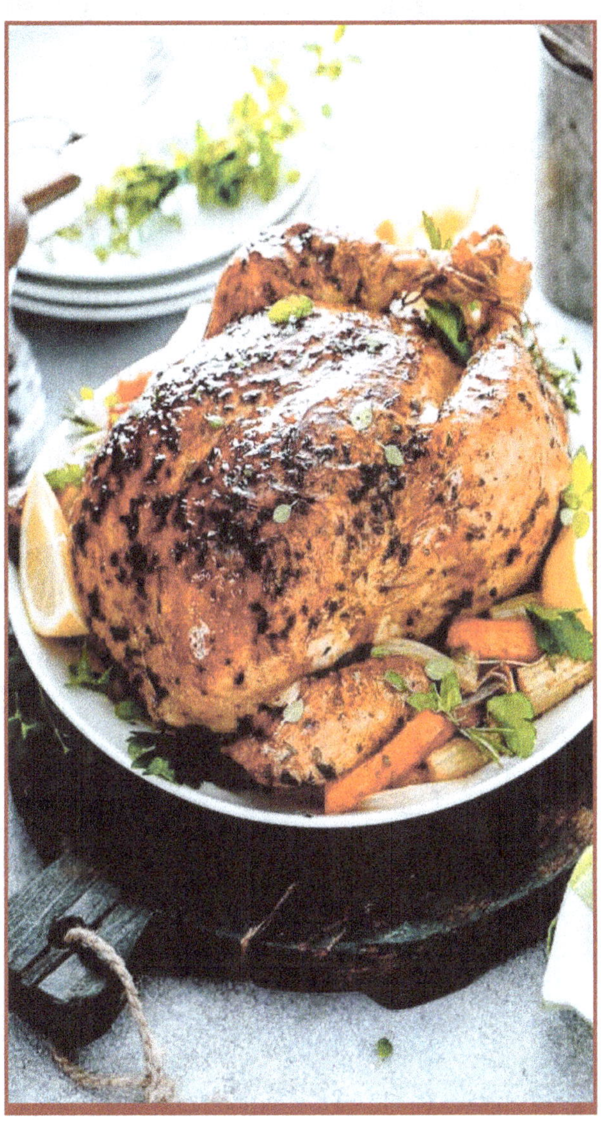

Time of Preparation: 10 minutes
Cooking Time: 20 minutes
Serving Unit: 2 servings

Ingredients:
- 2 boneless, skinless chicken breasts

- 2 cups mixed vegetables (such as bell peppers, carrots zucchini, and cherry tomatoes)
- 2 tablespoons olive oil
- 1 lemon, juiced and zested
- 2 cloves garlic, minced
- 1 teaspoon dried herbs (such as oregano, thyme, or rosemary)
- Salt and pepper to taste

Procedures:

1. Preheat your oven to 400°F (200°C).
2. Place the chicken breasts on a baking sheet lined with parchment paper or aluminum foil.
3. In a small bowl, whisk together the olive oil, lemon juice and zest, minced garlic, dried herbs, salt, and pepper.
4. Pour the marinade over the chicken breasts, making sure they are evenly coated. Set aside to marinate while you prepare the vegetables.
5. Chop the mixed vegetables into bite-sized pieces and place them in a large mixing bowl.
6. Drizzle olive oil over the vegetables and toss to coat. Season with salt, pepper, and any additional herbs or spices of your choice.
7. Spread the vegetables evenly around the chicken breasts on the baking sheet.
8. Roast in the preheated oven for 15-20 minutes, or until the chicken is cooked through and the vegetables are tender and slightly caramelized.
9. Remove from the oven and let the chicken rest for a few minutes before slicing.
10. Serve the lemon herb chicken alongside the roasted vegetables.

Cooking Tips:

- To ensure even cooking, try to cut the vegetables into uniform sizes so they roast evenly.
- Feel free to customize the vegetables based on your preferences and what's in season. Root vegetables like carrots and potatoes work well in this dish, as do green beans and broccoli.
- For extra flavor, you can add a sprinkle of grated Parmesan cheese over the vegetables during the last few minutes of roasting.
- If you prefer, you can grill the chicken and vegetables instead of roasting them in the oven. Simply preheat your grill to medium-high heat and cook the chicken for 6-7 minutes on each side, or until cooked through, and the vegetables for 8-10 minutes, or until tender.

Nutritional Values:

- Calories: Approximately 300 kcal per serving
- Protein: Approximately 25g per serving
- Carbohydrates: Approximately 15g per serving
- Fat: Approximately 15g per serving
- Fiber: Approximately 5g per serving

Health Benefits:

- Chicken is a lean source of protein that's rich in essential nutrients such as vitamins B6 and B12, niacin, phosphorus, and selenium, which support muscle growth and repair, immune function, and overall health.
- Mixed vegetables provide a variety of vitamins, minerals, and antioxidants, such as vitamins A, C, and K, folate, potassium, and fiber, which help reduce inflammation, support digestion, and promote overall health and wellbeing.

- Olive oil is rich in heart-healthy monounsaturated fats and antioxidants, such as oleic acid and polyphenols, which help reduce inflammation, support heart health, and improve cholesterol levels.
- Lemon juice and zest add a burst of flavor to the dish while providing vitamin C and antioxidants, which help boost immune function, support digestion, and detoxify the body.

Cabbage and Sausage Skillet

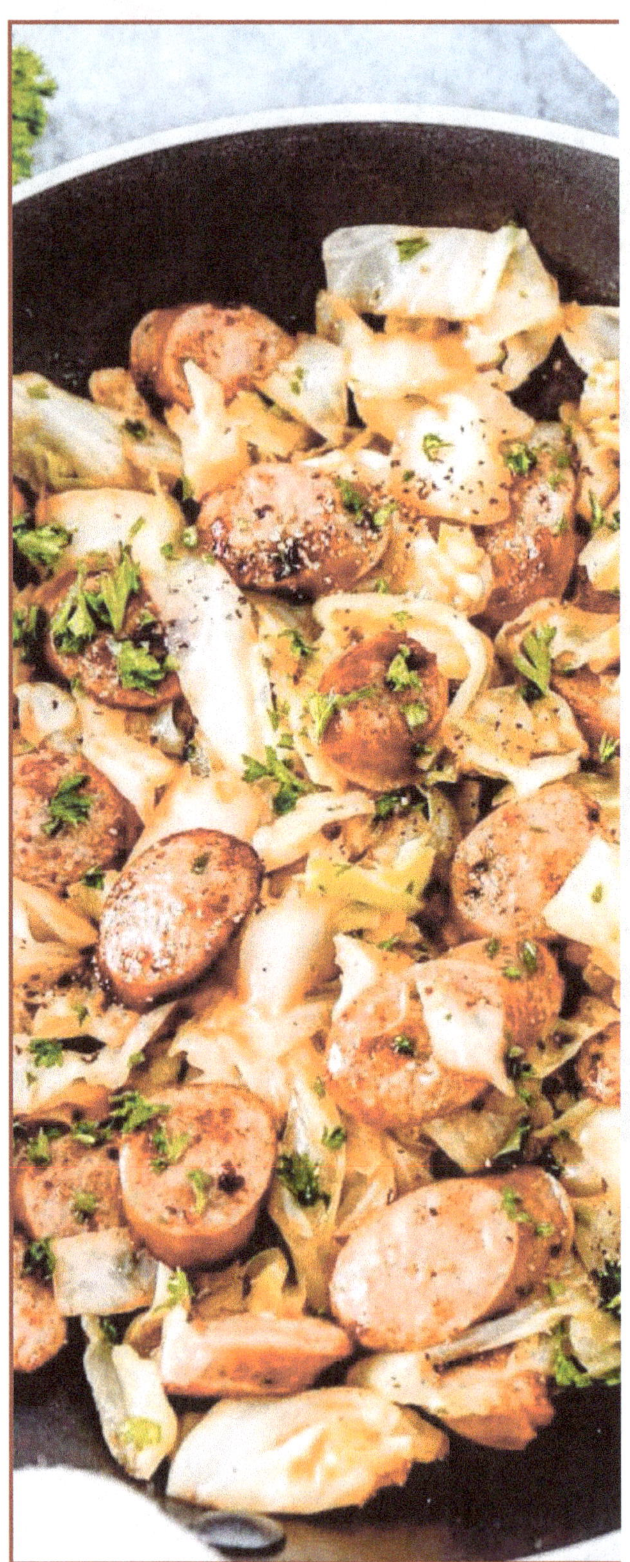

Time of Preparation: 10 minutes
Cooking Time: 20 minutes
Serving Unit: 4 servings

Ingredients:
- 1 pound smoked sausage, sliced (such as kielbasa or Andouille)
- 1 small head cabbage, thinly sliced
- 1 onion, thinly sliced
- 2 cloves garlic, minced
- 2 tablespoons olive oil
- Salt and pepper to taste

Procedures:
1. Heat olive oil in a large skillet or sauté pan over medium heat.
2. Add the sliced sausage to the skillet and cook for 5-6 minutes, stirring occasionally, until it is browned and heated through.
3. Once the sausage is cooked, remove it from the skillet and set it aside.
4. In the same skillet, add the thinly sliced cabbage and onion. Sauté for 5-7 minutes, stirring occasionally, until the vegetables are tender and caramelized.
5. Add the minced garlic to the skillet with the cabbage and onion, and sauté for an additional 1-2 minutes, until fragrant.
6. Return the cooked sausage to the skillet with the cabbage and onion mixture. Toss to combine everything evenly.
7. Season the Cabbage and Sausage Skillet with salt and pepper to taste, and adjust the seasoning according to your preference.
8. Remove the skillet from the heat and transfer the Cabbage and Sausage Skillet to a serving dish.
9. Serve immediately, and enjoy!

Cooking Tips:
- Choose smoked sausage such as kielbasa or Andouille for added

flavor, but feel free to use any type of sausage you prefer.
- Use a sharp knife to thinly slice the cabbage and onion for quicker cooking and better texture.
- Be sure to cook the cabbage until it's tender but still slightly crisp to maintain its texture and flavor.
- Customize the recipe by adding additional ingredients, such as diced bell peppers, carrots, or potatoes, for added flavor and variety.
- Serve the Cabbage and Sausage Skillet as a standalone meal or pair it with a side of rice, quinoa, or crusty bread for a complete and satisfying meal.

Nutritional Values:
- Calories: Approximately 300 kcal per serving
- Protein: Approximately 12g per serving
- Carbohydrates: Approximately 15g per serving
- Fat: Approximately 20g per serving
- Fiber: Approximately 6g per serving

Health Benefits:
- Cabbage is low in calories and carbohydrates but high in fiber, vitamins, and minerals, including vitamin C, vitamin K, and folate, which support digestive health, immune function, and bone health, and may help reduce the risk of chronic diseases.
- Smoked sausage is a good source of protein and fat, which provide energy and satiety, but choose leaner options and consume in moderation to minimize saturated fat and sodium intake.
- Onions and garlic add flavor and aroma to the dish, as well as vitamins, minerals, and antioxidants, including vitamin C, vitamin B6, and allicin, which support immune function, heart health, and inflammation reduction.
- Olive oil is rich in heart-healthy monounsaturated fats and antioxidants, including oleic acid and polyphenols, which may help reduce inflammation, lower cholesterol levels, and protect against heart disease and stroke.

Teriyaki Salmon with Broccoli

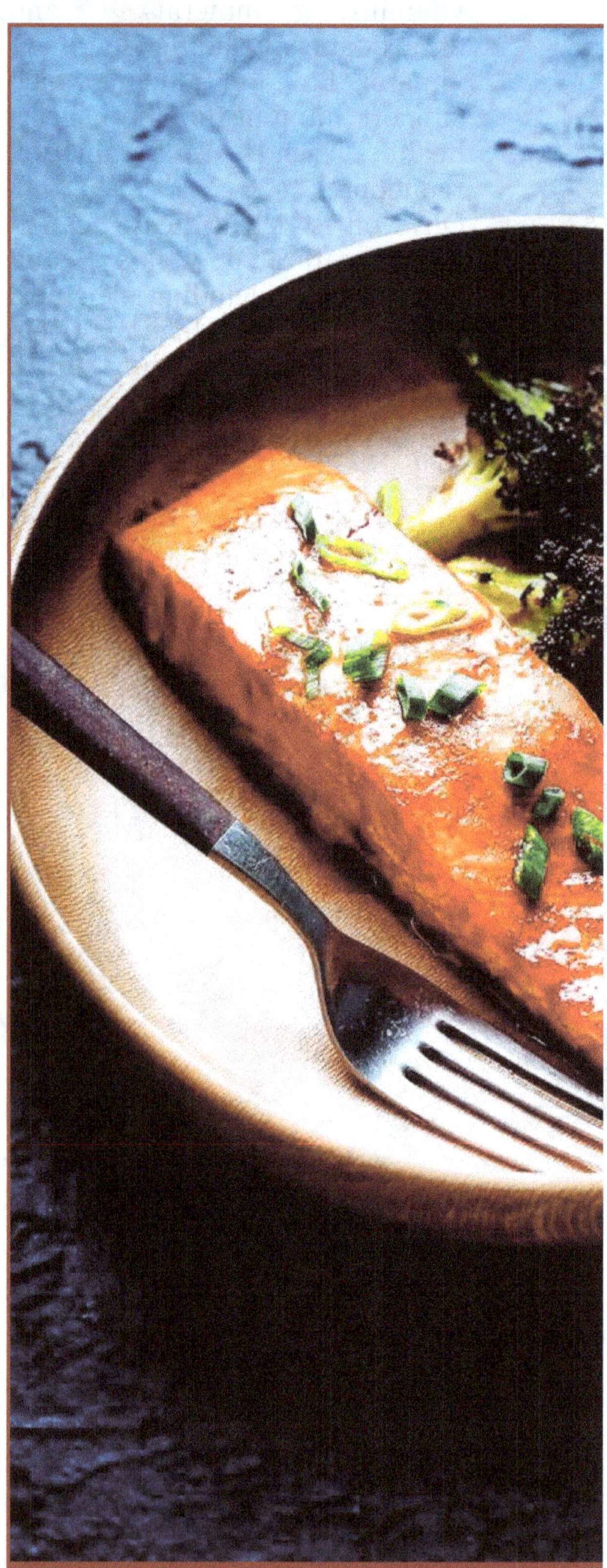

Time of Preparation: 10 minutes
Cooking Time: 15 minutes
Serving Unit: 2 servings

Ingredients:
- 2 salmon filets (about 6 ounces each)
- 2 cups broccoli florets
- 1/4 cup teriyaki sauce (store-bought or homemade)
- 2 tablespoons honey or maple syrup
- 1 tablespoon sesame seeds (optional)

Procedures:
1. Preheat your oven to 400°F (200°C).
2. Place the salmon fillets on a baking sheet lined with parchment paper or aluminum foil.
3. Arrange the broccoli florets around the salmon on the baking sheet.
4. In a small bowl, whisk together the teriyaki sauce and honey (or maple syrup) until well combined.
5. Pour the teriyaki sauce mixture over the salmon and broccoli, making sure they are evenly coated.
6. Sprinkle sesame seeds over the salmon fillets if desired.
7. Bake in the preheated oven for 12-15 minutes, or until the salmon is cooked through and flakes easily with a fork, and the broccoli is tender-crisp.
8. Remove from the oven and let it rest for a few minutes before serving.

Cooking Tips:
- For added flavor, you can marinate the salmon fillets in the teriyaki sauce mixture for 15-30 minutes before baking.
- Make sure to evenly coat the salmon and broccoli with the teriyaki sauce mixture to ensure they caramelize and develop a delicious glaze during baking.

- Keep an eye on the salmon while baking to prevent overcooking, as salmon can dry out quickly if cooked for too long.
- Serve the teriyaki salmon and broccoli with cooked rice or quinoa for a complete and satisfying meal.

Nutritional Values:
- Calories: Approximately 300 kcal per serving
- Protein: Approximately 25g per serving
- Carbohydrates: Approximately 20g per serving
- Fat: Approximately 15g per serving
- Fiber: Approximately 5g per serving

Health Benefits:
- Salmon is an excellent source of high-quality protein, omega-3 fatty acids, vitamins, and minerals, which support heart health, brain function, and overall wellbeing.
- Broccoli is a nutrient-dense vegetable that's rich in vitamins, minerals, and antioxidants, such as vitamin C, vitamin K, folate, and sulforaphane, which help reduce inflammation, support detoxification, and protect against chronic diseases.
- Teriyaki sauce provides a sweet and savory flavor to the dish while adding depth and complexity. Look for low-sodium or reduced-sugar teriyaki sauce options to keep the dish healthier.
- Honey or maple syrup adds natural sweetness to the teriyaki sauce without the need for refined sugars, providing a healthier alternative to traditional sweeteners.
- Sesame seeds are a good source of healthy fats, protein, and minerals, such as calcium, magnesium, and iron, which support bone health, energy production, and immune function.

Turkey and Sweet Potato Skillet

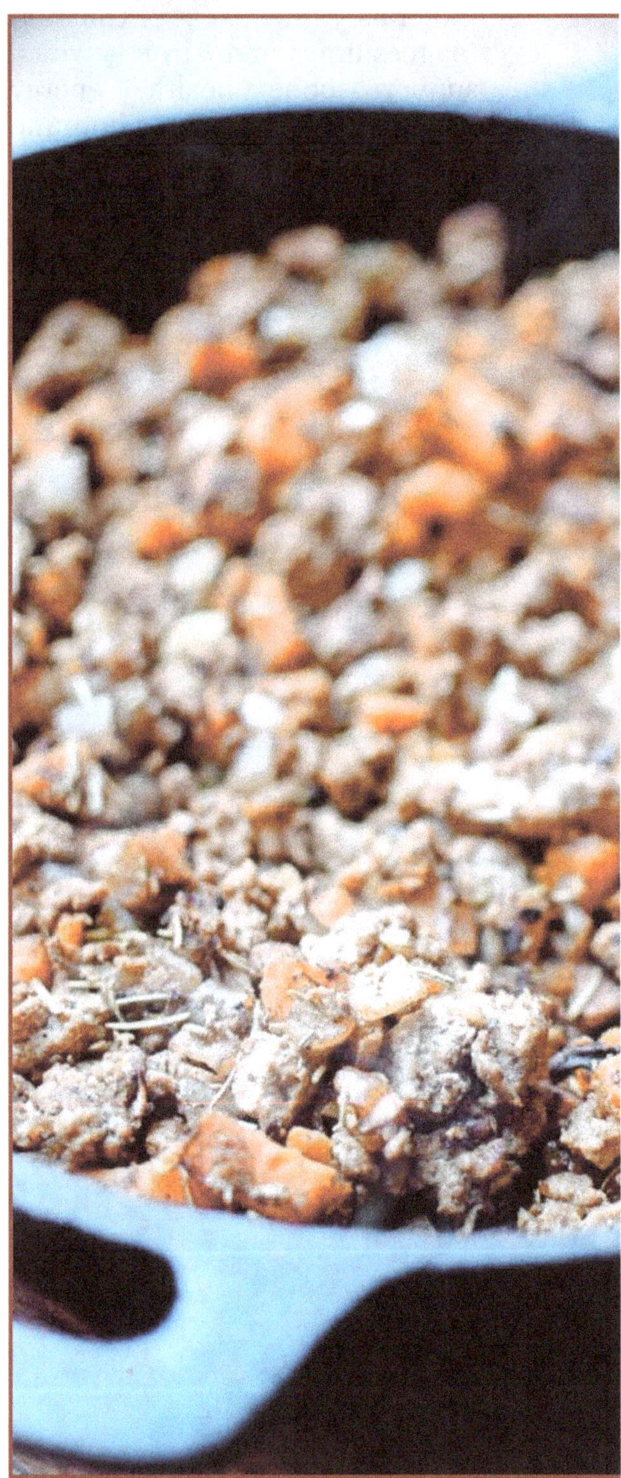

Time of Preparation: 10 minutes
Cooking Time: 20 minutes
Serving Unit: 2 servings

Ingredients:

- 1 pound ground turkey
- 2 medium sweet potatoes, peeled and diced
- 1 onion, diced
- 2 cloves garlic, minced
- 1 tablespoon olive oil
- Salt and pepper to taste

Procedures:

1. Heat olive oil in a large skillet over medium heat.
2. Add diced sweet potatoes to the skillet and cook for about 5 minutes, stirring occasionally, until they begin to soften.
3. Add diced onion to the skillet and cook for another 3-4 minutes, until the onion is translucent.
4. Add minced garlic to the skillet and cook for an additional 1-2 minutes, until fragrant.
5. Push the sweet potatoes, onion, and garlic to one side of the skillet, and add ground turkey to the other side.
6. Cook the ground turkey, breaking it apart with a spoon, until it is no longer pink and fully cooked.
7. Stir the cooked turkey into the sweet potato mixture, and season with salt and pepper to taste.
8. Cook for another 2-3 minutes, until everything is heated through and well combined.
9. Serve the turkey and sweet potato skillet hot, garnished with fresh herbs if desired.

Cooking Tips:

- To save time, you can use pre-cooked or leftover sweet potatoes instead of peeling and dicing them from scratch.

- Feel free to customize the skillet with additional vegetables such as bell peppers, spinach, or kale for added flavor and nutrition.
- For extra flavor, you can season the skillet with your favorite herbs and spices such as paprika, cumin, or chili powder.
- Serve the turkey and sweet potato skillet with a side of steamed vegetables or a simple salad for a complete and balanced meal.

Nutritional Values:
- Calories: Approximately 300 kcal per serving
- Protein: Approximately 25g per serving
- Carbohydrates: Approximately 20g per serving
- Fat: Approximately 15g per serving
- Fiber: Approximately 4g per serving

Health Benefits:
- Ground turkey is a lean source of protein that's lower in fat and calories compared to other meats, making it a healthier option for weight management and heart health.
- Sweet potatoes are rich in vitamins, minerals, and antioxidants, such as vitamin A, vitamin C, potassium, and beta-carotene, which help support immune function, regulate blood sugar levels, and promote healthy vision.
- Onions and garlic are rich in sulfur compounds and antioxidants, which help reduce inflammation, support immune function, and protect against chronic diseases.
- Olive oil provides heart-healthy monounsaturated fats and antioxidants, such as oleic acid and polyphenols, which help reduce inflammation, support heart health, and improve cholesterol levels.

Sautéed Spinach and White Beans

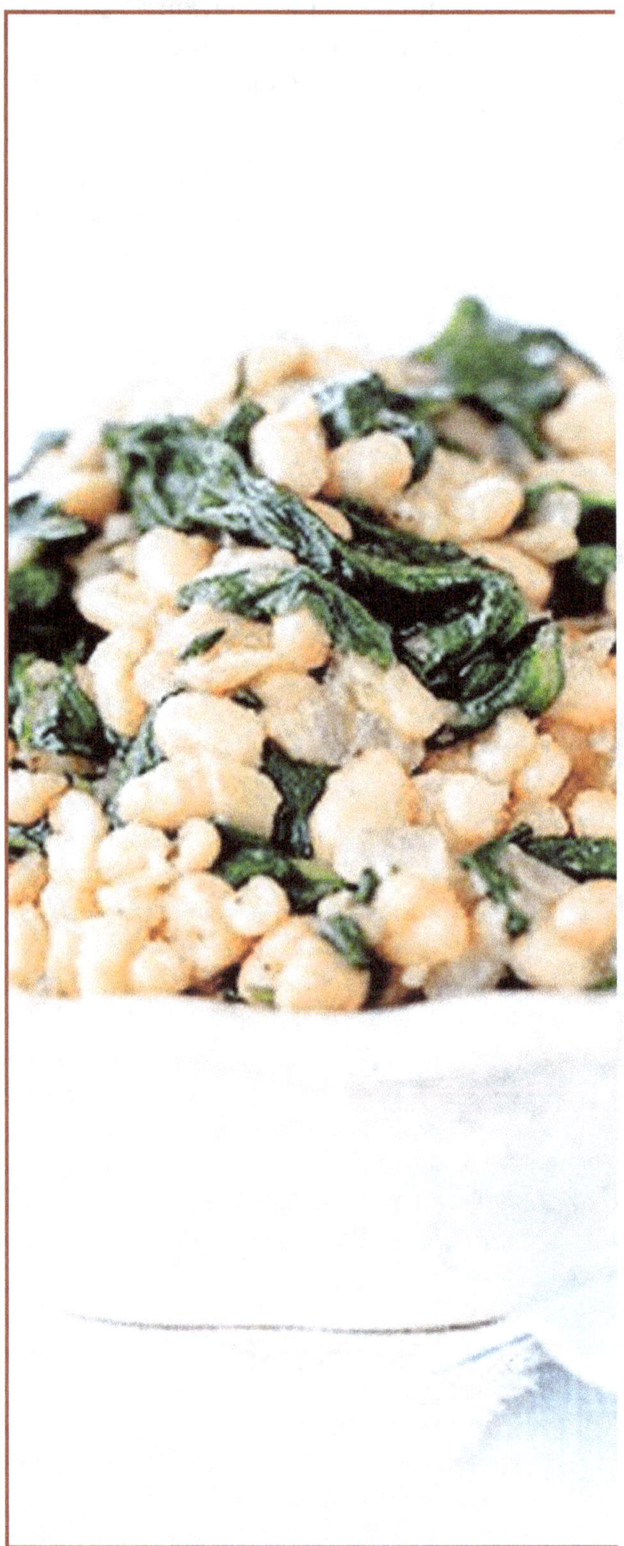

Time of Preparation: 5 minutes
Cooking Time: 10 minutes
Serving Unit: 2 servings

Ingredients:
- 6 cups fresh spinach leaves
- 1 can (15 ounces) white beans, drained and rinsed
- 2 cloves garlic, minced
- 2 tablespoons olive oil
- Salt and pepper to taste
- Lemon wedges for serving (optional)

Procedures:
1. Heat olive oil in a large skillet over medium heat.
2. Add minced garlic to the skillet and sauté for 1 minute, until fragrant.
3. Add the fresh spinach leaves to the skillet and cook, stirring occasionally, for 2-3 minutes, until wilted.
4. Add the drained and rinsed white beans to the skillet and stir to combine with the spinach.
5. Season with salt and pepper to taste and continue cooking for an additional 2-3 minutes, until the beans are heated through.
6. Remove the skillet from the heat and transfer the sautéed spinach and white beans to a serving dish.
7. Serve immediately, with lemon wedges on the side for squeezing over the dish, if desired.

Cooking Tips:
- Be sure not to overcrowd the skillet when cooking the spinach. Cook in batches if necessary to ensure even wilting.
- Feel free to customize the recipe with additional ingredients, such as diced onions, cherry tomatoes,

or red pepper flakes for added flavor and texture.

- Serve the sautéed spinach and white beans as a side dish or as a main course with crusty bread or cooked grains, such as quinoa or rice.

Nutritional Values:

- Calories: Approximately 200 kcal per serving
- Protein: Approximately 10g per serving
- Carbohydrates: Approximately 20g per serving
- Fat: Approximately 10g per serving
- Fiber: Approximately 8g per serving

Health Benefits:

- Spinach is rich in vitamins A, C, and K, as well as iron, calcium, and antioxidants, which support overall health and immune function.
- White beans are an excellent source of protein, fiber, and complex carbohydrates, which help promote satiety, regulate blood sugar levels, and support digestive health.
- Garlic contains sulfur compounds with anti-inflammatory and immune-boosting properties, as well as antioxidants that help protect against chronic diseases.
- Olive oil is rich in heart-healthy monounsaturated fats and antioxidants, which may help reduce the risk of heart disease and inflammation.
- This dish is low in calories and saturated fat, making it a nutritious and satisfying option for individuals looking to maintain a healthy weight or manage diabetes.

Veggie-Packed Quinoa Stir-Fry

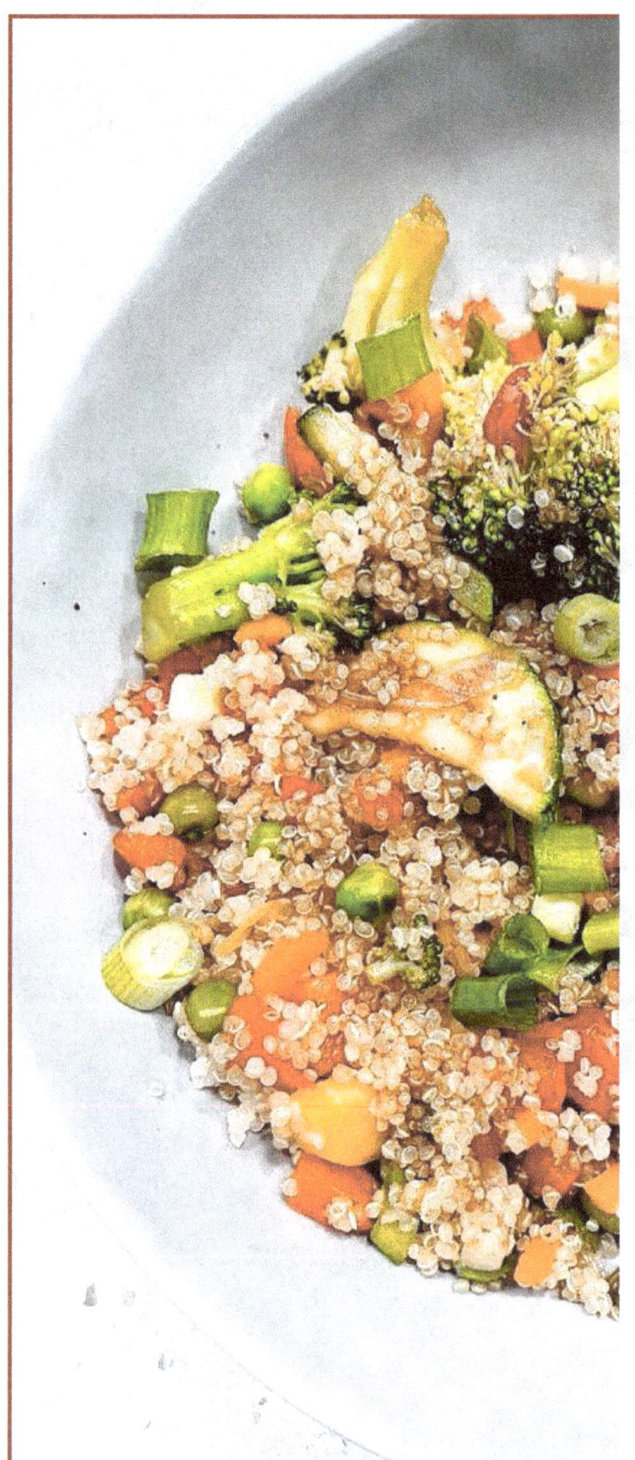

Time of Preparation: 10 minutes
Cooking Time: 20 minutes
Serving Unit: 2 servings

Ingredients:
- 1 cup quinoa, rinsed and drained
- 2 cups mixed vegetables (such as bell peppers, tomatoes, cucumber carrots, broccoli, and snap peas)
- 2 tablespoons soy sauce or tamari
- 1 tablespoon sesame oil
- 2 cloves garlic, minced
- Optional toppings: sliced green onions, sesame seeds, crushed red pepper flakes

Procedures:
1. Cook quinoa according to package instructions. Once cooked, fluff with a fork and set aside.
2. Heat sesame oil in a large skillet or wok over medium heat.
3. Add minced garlic to the skillet and cook for 1 minute until fragrant.
4. Add mixed vegetables to the skillet and stir-fry for 5-7 minutes until tender-crisp.
5. Add cooked quinoa to the skillet, followed by soy sauce or tamari.
6. Stir-fry everything together for another 2-3 minutes until the quinoa is heated through and well coated with the sauce.
7. Remove from heat and divide the stir-fry between two serving plates.
8. Garnish with sliced green onions, sesame seeds, and crushed red pepper flakes if desired.
9. Serve hot and enjoy!

Cooking Tips:
- Feel free to customize the stir-fry with your favorite vegetables or whatever you have on hand. Other great options include mushrooms, cabbage, snow peas, or baby corn.

- To save time, you can use pre-cut or frozen mixed vegetables instead of chopping them yourself.
- For added protein, you can add cooked chicken, tofu, or edamame to the stir-fry.
- Make sure to rinse the quinoa before cooking to remove any bitterness or residue.
- Use low-sodium soy sauce or tamari to reduce the sodium content of the stir-fry.
- To make the stir-fry gluten-free, use tamari instead of soy sauce.

Nutritional Values:
- Calories: Approximately 300 kcal per serving
- Protein: Approximately 10g per serving
- Carbohydrates: Approximately 50g per serving
- Fat: Approximately 8g per serving
- Fiber: Approximately 8g per serving

Health Benefits:
- Quinoa is a complete protein source, meaning it contains all nine essential amino acids, making it an excellent plant-based protein option for vegetarians and vegans. It's also high in fiber, vitamins, and minerals, such as magnesium, iron, and manganese, which support digestion, heart health, and overall wellbeing.
- Mixed vegetables provide a variety of vitamins, minerals, and antioxidants, such as vitamins A, C, and K, folate, potassium, and fiber, which help reduce inflammation, support immune function, and promote overall health and wellbeing.
- Soy sauce or tamari adds flavor to the stir-fry while providing essential amino acids and minerals such as iron and potassium.
- Sesame oil adds a rich, nutty flavor to the stir-fry and is rich in heart-healthy monounsaturated fats, vitamins, and antioxidants, such as vitamin E and sesamol, which help reduce inflammation, support heart health, and improve cholesterol levels.

Chapter 5: Nourishing Soups and Stews

Chapter 5: Nourishing Soups and Stews

Welcome to Chapter 5, where we explore nourishing soups and stews that are both comforting and nutritious. In this chapter, I'll delve into a variety of recipes that are perfect for cozy evenings or chilly days, providing warmth and satisfaction while also supporting your health and wellbeing.

From hearty vegetable soups to protein-packed stews, these recipes are designed to nourish your body with wholesome ingredients while also being quick and easy to prepare. Whether you're craving a classic chicken noodle soup, a spicy chili, or a creamy pumpkin bisque, you'll find plenty of inspiration in this chapter to keep you warm and satisfied all season long. Let's get cooking and enjoy the comforting goodness of homemade soups and stews!

Hearty Lentil Soup

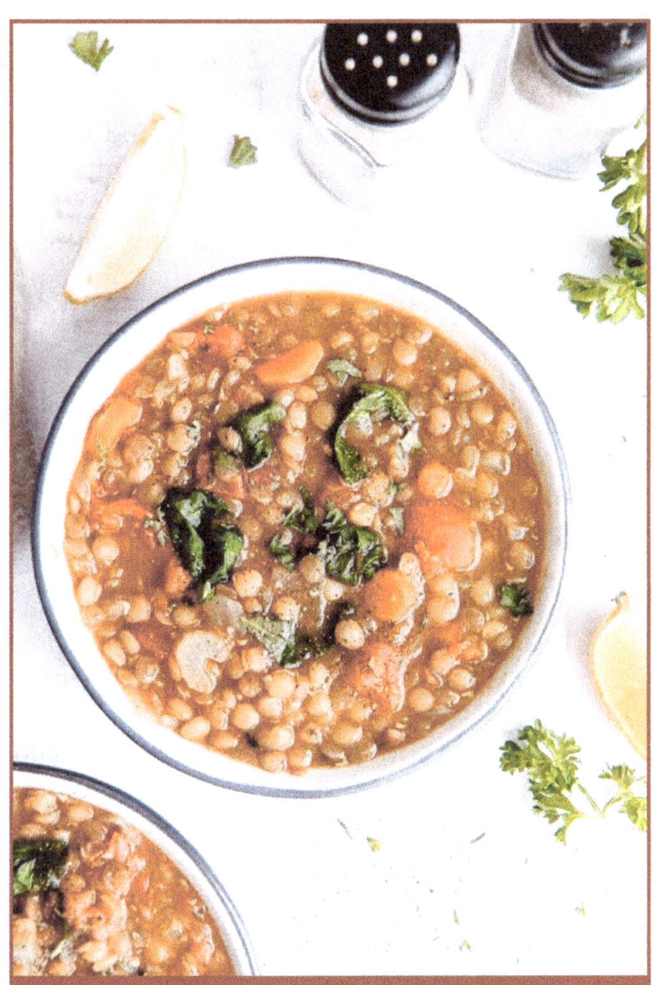

Time of Preparation: 10 minutes
Cooking Time: 20 minutes
Serving Unit: 4 servings

Ingredients:
- 1 cup dried green or brown lentils, rinsed and drained
- 1 onion, diced
- 2 carrots, diced
- 2 stalks celery, diced
- 4 cups vegetable broth
- 2 cloves garlic, minced
- 1 teaspoon ground cumin

- 1 teaspoon ground turmeric
- Salt and pepper to taste
- Optional toppings: chopped fresh parsley, lemon wedges, Greek yogurt

Procedures:

1. In a large pot or Dutch oven, heat olive oil over medium heat.
2. Add diced onion, carrots, and celery to the pot and sauté for 5-7 minutes until softened.
3. Add minced garlic, ground cumin, and ground turmeric to the pot and sauté for another 1-2 minutes until fragrant.
4. Add rinsed lentils and vegetable broth to the pot. Bring to a boil, then reduce heat to low and simmer for 15-20 minutes until the lentils are tender.
5. Season the soup with salt and pepper to taste.
6. If desired, use an immersion blender to partially blend the soup for a thicker consistency, leaving some lentils whole for texture.
7. Serve hot, garnished with chopped fresh parsley and a squeeze of lemon juice if desired. You can also add a dollop of Greek yogurt for extra creaminess.

Cooking Tips:

- To save time, you can use pre-cut or frozen diced vegetables instead of chopping them yourself.
- Rinse the lentils under cold water before cooking to remove any debris or dust.
- Feel free to customize the soup with additional vegetables or spices according to your taste preferences. You can add diced potatoes, chopped spinach, or diced tomatoes for extra flavor and nutrition.

- For added protein, you can add cooked chicken, turkey, or sausage to the soup.

Nutritional Values:

- Calories: Approximately 200 kcal per serving
- Protein: Approximately 10g per serving
- Carbohydrates: Approximately 35g per serving
- Fat: Approximately 1g per serving
- Fiber: Approximately 10g per serving

Health Benefits:

- Lentils are a nutritional powerhouse, packed with protein, fiber, vitamins, and minerals, such as folate, iron, and potassium, which support heart health, digestion, and overall wellbeing.
- Vegetables such as onions, carrots, and celery are rich in vitamins, minerals, and antioxidants, which help reduce inflammation, support immune function, and promote healthy digestion.
- Garlic contains sulfur compounds and antioxidants, such as allicin and quercetin, which have antibacterial and anti-inflammatory properties and help boost immune function and protect against chronic diseases.
- Spices such as cumin and turmeric provide flavor and aroma to the soup while also offering health benefits. Cumin aids digestion and may help improve blood sugar control, while turmeric contains curcumin, a powerful antioxidant with anti-inflammatory properties.

Creamy Tomato Basil Soup

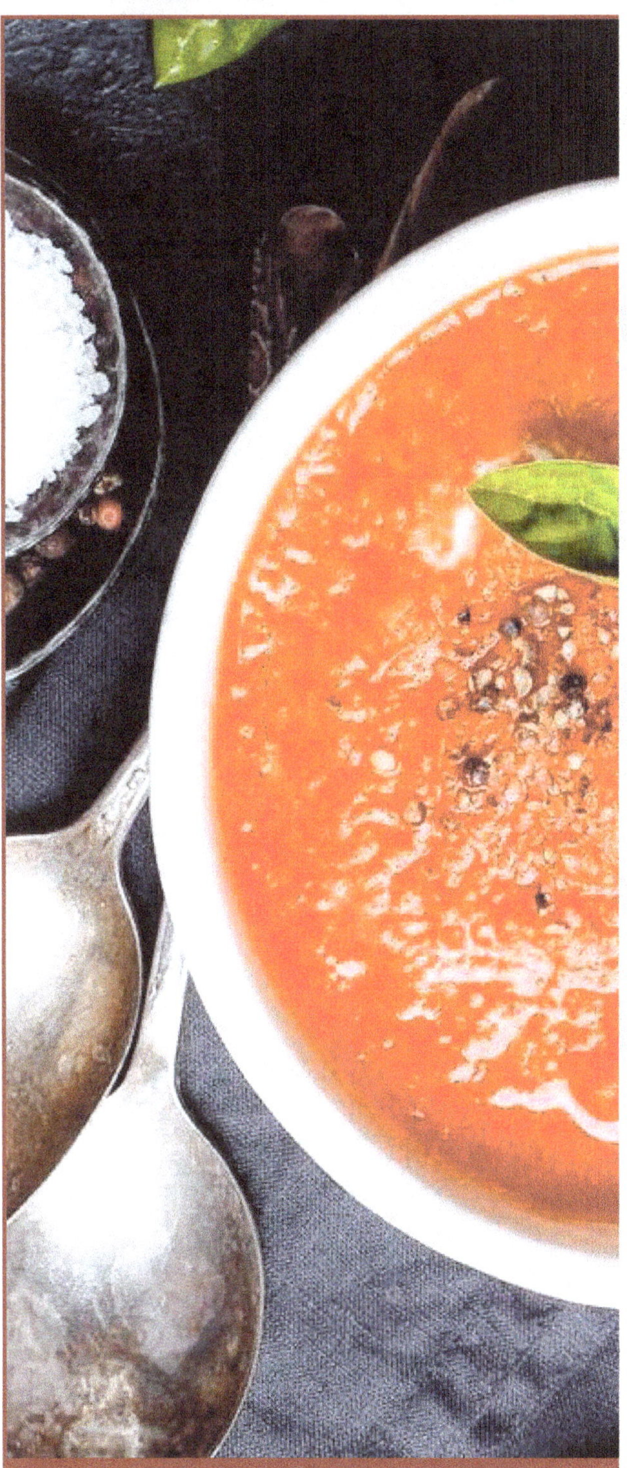

Time of Preparation: 10 minutes
Cooking Time: 20 minutes
Serving Unit: 4 servings

Ingredients:

- 2 cans (14 oz each) diced tomatoes
- 1 onion, diced
- 2 cloves garlic, minced
- 1 cup vegetable broth
- 1/2 cup heavy cream or coconut cream
- Handful of fresh basil leaves, chopped (plus extra for garnish)
- Salt and pepper to taste
- Optional toppings: grated Parmesan cheese, croutons, drizzle of olive oil

Procedures:

1. In a large pot or Dutch oven, heat olive oil over medium heat.

2. Add diced onion to the pot and sauté for 5-7 minutes until softened.

3. Add minced garlic to the pot and sauté for another 1-2 minutes until fragrant.

4. Add diced tomatoes (with their juices) to the pot, along with vegetable broth and chopped basil leaves. Bring to a simmer.

5. Reduce heat to low and let the soup simmer for 10-15 minutes to allow the flavors to meld together.

6. Use an immersion blender to blend the soup until smooth and creamy. Alternatively, you can transfer the soup to a blender and blend in batches until smooth, then return to the pot.

7. Stir in heavy cream or coconut cream until well combined. Season with salt and pepper to taste.

8. Serve hot, garnished with additional chopped basil leaves and your choice of toppings.

Cooking Tips:

- For extra flavor, you can roast the diced tomatoes in the oven before adding them to the soup. Simply toss the tomatoes with olive oil, salt, and pepper, and roast at 400°F (200°C) for 20-25 minutes until caramelized.
- If you prefer a chunkier soup, you can leave some of the diced tomatoes unblended.
- To make the soup dairy-free and vegan, use coconut cream instead of heavy cream.
- Serve the soup with a side of crusty bread or grilled cheese sandwiches for a satisfying meal.

Nutritional Values:

Calories: Approximately 200 kcal per serving
Protein: Approximately 4g per serving
Carbohydrates: Approximately 20g per serving
Fat: Approximately 12g per serving
Fiber: Approximately 5g per serving

Health Benefits:

- Tomatoes are rich in vitamins, minerals, and antioxidants, such as vitamin C, potassium, and lycopene, which help reduce inflammation, support heart health, and protect against certain types of cancer.
- Onions and garlic contain sulfur compounds and antioxidants, such as allicin and quercetin, which have antibacterial and anti-inflammatory properties and help boost immune function and protect against chronic diseases.
- Basil is a fragrant herb that's rich in vitamins A, K, and C, as well as antioxidants, which help reduce inflammation, support digestion, and promote overall health and wellbeing.
- Vegetable broth provides flavor and depth to the soup without adding extra calories or fat, making it a healthy alternative to store-bought broths that may be high in sodium and preservatives.
- Heavy cream or coconut cream adds richness and creaminess to the soup while also providing essential fats and calories for energy and satiety.

Chunky Vegetable Beef Stew

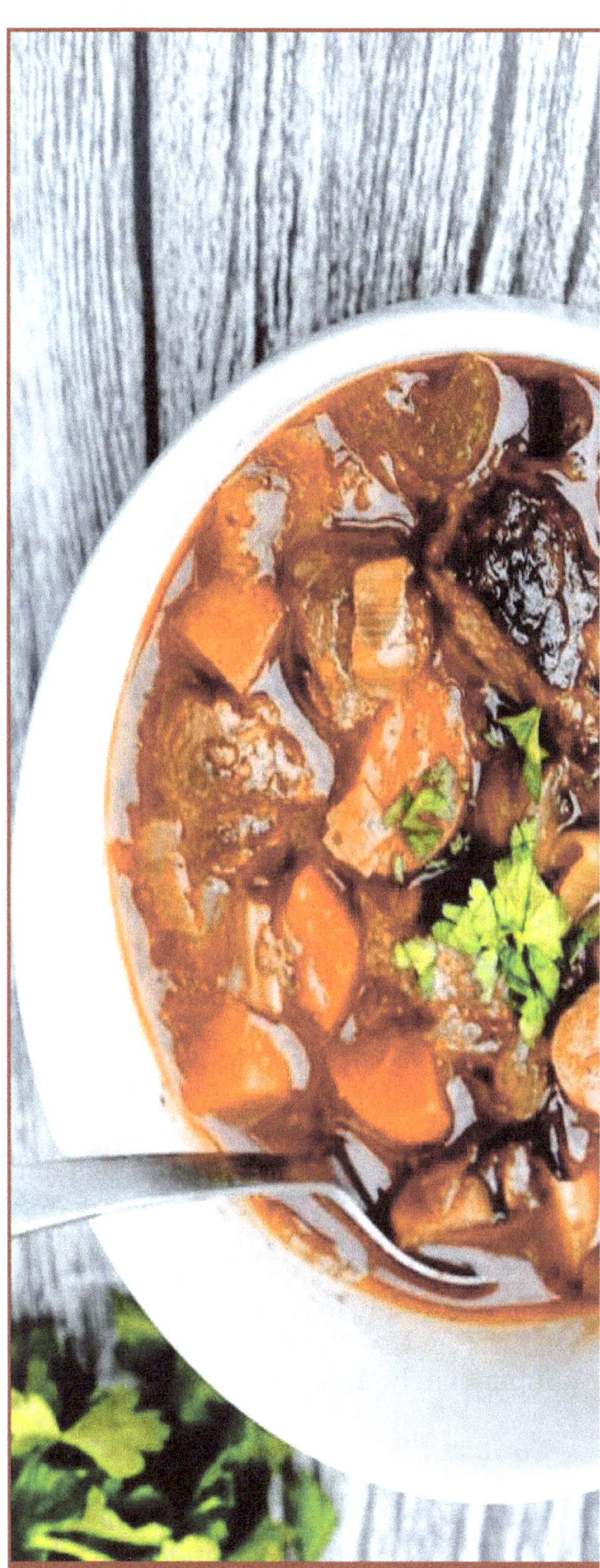

Time of Preparation: 10 minutes
Cooking Time: 20 minutes
Serving Unit: 4 servings

Ingredients:
- 1 pound beef stew meat, cubed
- 2 cups mixed vegetables (such as carrots, potatoes, green beans, and peas)
- 1 onion, diced
- 2 cloves garlic, minced
- 4 cups beef broth
- Salt and pepper to taste

Procedures:
1. In a large pot or Dutch oven, heat olive oil over medium-high heat.
2. Add cubed beef stew meat to the pot and cook until browned on all sides, about 5-7 minutes.
3. Add diced onion to the pot and sauté for 2-3 minutes until softened.
4. Add minced garlic to the pot and sauté for another 1-2 minutes until fragrant.
5. Add mixed vegetables and beef broth to the pot. Bring to a boil.
6. Reduce heat to low, cover, and let the stew simmer for 15-20 minutes until the vegetables are tender and the beef is cooked through.
7. Season with salt and pepper to taste.
8. Serve hot, garnished with fresh herbs if desired.

Cooking Tips:
- To save time, you can use pre-cut or frozen mixed vegetables instead of chopping them yourself.
- For extra flavor, you can add herbs and spices such as thyme, rosemary, or bay leaves to the stew.
- If you prefer a thicker stew, you can mix a tablespoon of

cornstarch with water and stir it into the stew during the last few minutes of cooking to thicken the broth.
- Serve the stew with a side of crusty bread or mashed potatoes for a hearty and satisfying meal.

Nutritional Values:
- Calories: Approximately 300 kcal per serving
- Protein: Approximately 25g per serving
- Carbohydrates: Approximately 20g per serving
- Fat: Approximately 10g per serving
- Fiber: Approximately 5g per serving

Health Benefits:
- Beef stew meat is a good source of protein, iron, and B vitamins, which help support muscle growth, energy production, and overall health and wellbeing.
- Mixed vegetables provide a variety of vitamins, minerals, and antioxidants, such as vitamin A, vitamin C, potassium, and fiber, which help reduce inflammation, support immune function, and promote healthy digestion.
- Onions and garlic contain sulfur compounds and antioxidants, such as allicin and quercetin, which have antibacterial and anti-inflammatory properties and help boost immune function and protect against chronic diseases.
- Beef broth provides flavor and depth to the stew without adding extra calories or fat, making it a healthy alternative to store-bought broths that may be high in sodium and preservatives.

Pesto Zucchini Noodles

Time of Preparation: 10 minutes
Cooking Time: 5 minutes
Serving Unit: 2 servings

Ingredients:
- 2 medium zucchini
- 1/4 cup basil pesto (homemade or store-bought)
- 1 tablespoon olive oil
- 2 tablespoons grated Parmesan cheese
- Salt and pepper to taste

Procedures:
1. Using a spiralizer or vegetable peeler, spiralize or julienne the zucchini into noodles. Alternatively, you can use a knife to thinly slice the zucchini lengthwise into strips resembling noodles.
2. Heat olive oil in a large skillet over medium heat.
3. Add the zucchini noodles to the skillet and sauté for 2-3 minutes, stirring occasionally, until they are just tender but still crisp.
4. Add the basil pesto to the skillet with the zucchini noodles and toss to coat evenly.
5. Cook for an additional 1-2 minutes, until the pesto is heated through and the zucchini noodles are well coated.
6. Remove the skillet from the heat and sprinkle grated Parmesan cheese over the pesto zucchini noodles.
7. Season with salt and pepper to taste and toss gently to combine.
8. Serve the Pesto Zucchini Noodles immediately, and enjoy!

Cooking Tips:
- Be careful not to overcook the zucchini noodles, as they can become mushy and lose their

texture. Cook them just until they are tender but still firm to the bite.

- If you prefer softer noodles, you can cover the skillet with a lid while cooking to steam the zucchini noodles.
- Customize the recipe by adding additional ingredients, such as cherry tomatoes, pine nuts, or grilled chicken, for added flavor and texture.
- Feel free to use homemade or store-bought basil pesto, depending on your preference and availability.

Nutritional Values:
- Calories: Approximately 150 kcal per serving
- Protein: Approximately 3g per serving
- Carbohydrates: Approximately 8g per serving
- Fat: Approximately 12g per serving
- Fiber: Approximately 2g per serving

Health Benefits:
- Zucchini is low in calories and carbohydrates but high in vitamins, minerals, and antioxidants, including vitamin C, vitamin K, and potassium, which support immune function, bone health, and heart health.
- Basil pesto is made with fresh basil leaves, garlic, olive oil, pine nuts, and Parmesan cheese, providing vitamins, minerals, and healthy fats that promote overall health and well-being.
- Olive oil is rich in heart-healthy monounsaturated fats and antioxidants, which may help reduce the risk of heart disease, inflammation, and oxidative stress.
- Parmesan cheese adds flavor and creaminess to the dish, but you can use a smaller amount or opt for a lower-fat cheese alternative to reduce saturated fat intake.
- This dish is low in calories and carbohydrates but rich in flavor, making it a satisfying option for individuals looking to manage their weight or blood sugar levels.

Chicken and Vegetable Noodle Soup

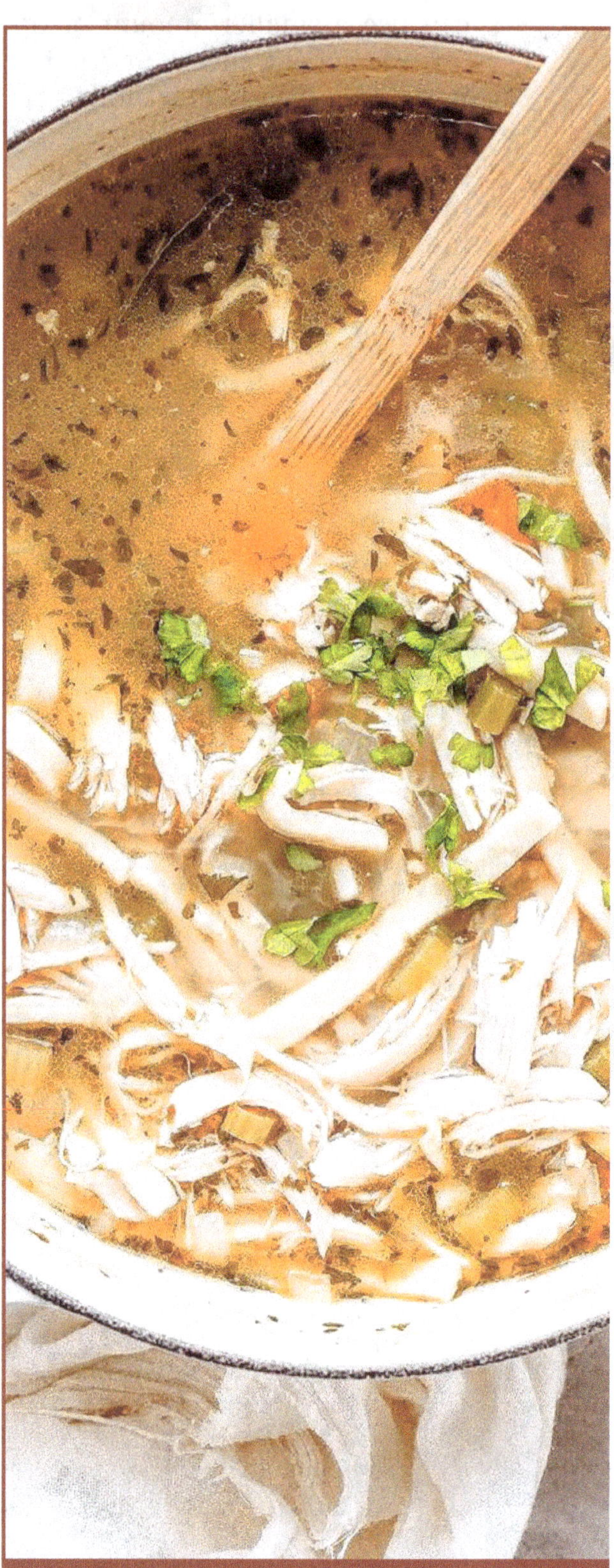

Time of Preparation: 10 minutes
Cooking Time: 20 minutes
Serving Unit: 4 servings

Ingredients:
- 8 cups chicken broth
- 2 cups cooked chicken breast, shredded
- 2 cups mixed vegetables (such as carrots, celery, and peas)
- 1 onion, diced
- 4 oz egg noodles
- Salt and pepper to taste

Procedures:

1. In a large pot or Dutch oven, bring chicken broth to a boil over medium-high heat.
2. Add diced onion to the pot and simmer for 5-7 minutes until softened.
3. Add mixed vegetables to the pot and cook for another 5 minutes until tender.
4. Add shredded chicken breast and egg noodles to the pot and cook for 8-10 minutes until the noodles are al dente and the chicken is heated through.
5. Season with salt and pepper to taste.
6. Serve hot, garnished with chopped fresh herbs if desired.

Cooking Tips:
- To save time, you can use pre-cooked or rotisserie chicken breast instead of cooking it from scratch.
- For extra flavor, you can add herbs and spices such as thyme, rosemary, or bay leaves to the soup.
- If you prefer a thicker soup, you can mix a tablespoon of cornstarch with water and stir it into the soup during the last few

minutes of cooking to thicken the broth.

- Feel free to customize the soup with additional vegetables or noodles according to your taste preferences. You can add spinach, kale, or mushrooms for extra flavor and nutrition.
- Serve the soup with a side of crusty bread or crackers for a complete and satisfying meal.

Nutritional Values:

- Calories: Approximately 250 kcal per serving
- Protein: Approximately 20g per serving
- Carbohydrates: Approximately 25g per serving
- Fat: Approximately 8g per serving
- Fiber: Approximately 4g per serving

Health Benefits:

- Chicken broth provides flavor and depth to the soup without adding extra calories or fat, making it a healthy base for the soup.
- Cooked chicken breast is a lean source of protein that's low in fat and calories, making it a healthy addition to the soup.
- Mixed vegetables provide a variety of vitamins, minerals, and antioxidants, such as vitamin A, vitamin C, potassium, and fiber, which help reduce inflammation, support immune function, and promote healthy digestion.
- Egg noodles are a good source of carbohydrates, which provide energy for the body, while also adding texture and bulk to the soup.

Chapter 6: Flavorful Fish and Seafood

Chapter 6: Flavorful Fish and Seafood

Welcome to Chapter 6, where we explore flavorful fish and seafood recipes that are not only delicious but also beneficial for your health. In this chapter, I'll dive into a variety of dishes featuring fresh fish and seafood, from simple grilled salmon to zesty shrimp tacos.

Fish and seafood are excellent sources of protein, omega-3 fatty acids, vitamins, and minerals, making them a nutritious addition to any diet. Whether you're a seafood enthusiast or looking to incorporate more healthy proteins into your meals, you'll find plenty of inspiration in this chapter to tantalize your taste buds and support your well-being. Let's embark on a culinary journey through the bountiful flavors of fish and seafood!

Honey Mustard Glazed Salmon

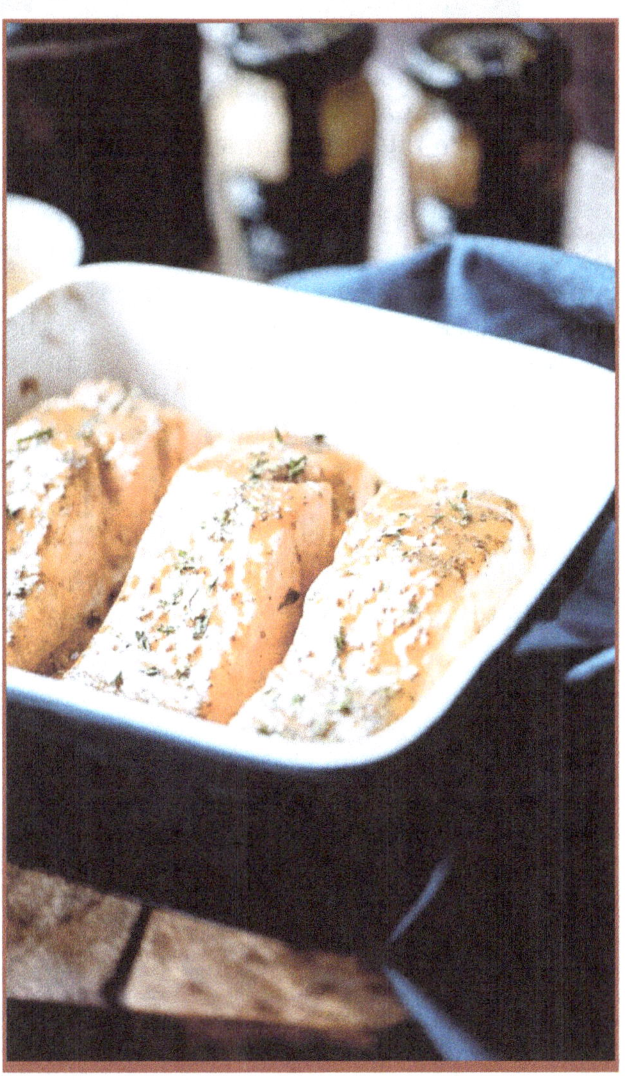

Time of Preparation: 5 minutes
Cooking Time: 15 minutes
Serving Unit: 2 servings

Ingredients:
- 2 salmon fillets (6 ounces each), skin-on or skinless
- 2 tablespoons honey
- 2 tablespoons Dijon mustard

- 1 tablespoon olive oil
- Salt and pepper to taste

Procedures:

1. Preheat your oven to 400°F (200°C).
2. In a small bowl, whisk together the honey, Dijon mustard, and olive oil until well combined.
3. Place the salmon fillets on a baking sheet lined with parchment paper or aluminum foil.
4. Season the salmon fillets with salt and pepper to taste.
5. Brush the honey mustard glaze evenly over the top of each salmon fillet, coating them generously.
6. Place the baking sheet in the preheated oven and bake for 12-15 minutes, or until the salmon is cooked through and flakes easily with a fork.
7. Remove the salmon from the oven and let it rest for a few minutes before serving.
8. Serve the Honey Mustard Glazed Salmon immediately, and enjoy!

Cooking Tips:

- Choose salmon fillets that are similar in size and thickness for even cooking.
- If using salmon fillets with the skin on, place them skin-side down on the baking sheet to prevent sticking.
- To prevent the honey mustard glaze from burning, you can cover the salmon loosely with aluminum foil during the first half of the baking time, then remove the foil for the remaining cooking time to allow the glaze to caramelize.
- For a stronger mustard flavor, you can add more Dijon mustard to the glaze mixture, according to your preference.

Nutritional Values:

- Calories: Approximately 300 kcal per serving
- Protein: Approximately 30g per serving
- Carbohydrates: Approximately 15g per serving
- Fat: Approximately 15g per serving
- Fiber: Approximately 0g per serving

Health Benefits:

- Salmon is rich in omega-3 fatty acids, which are essential fats that support heart health, brain function, and inflammation reduction.
- Honey is a natural sweetener that provides energy and antioxidants, but use it in moderation to avoid excessive sugar intake.
- Dijon mustard adds tanginess and depth of flavor to the glaze, as well as vitamins, minerals, and antioxidants that support overall health and well-being.
- Olive oil is rich in heart-healthy monounsaturated fats and antioxidants, which may help reduce the risk of heart disease and inflammation.
- This dish is low in carbohydrates but high in protein and healthy fats, making it a nutritious and satisfying option for individuals looking to manage their weight or blood sugar levels.

Garlic Butter Shrimp

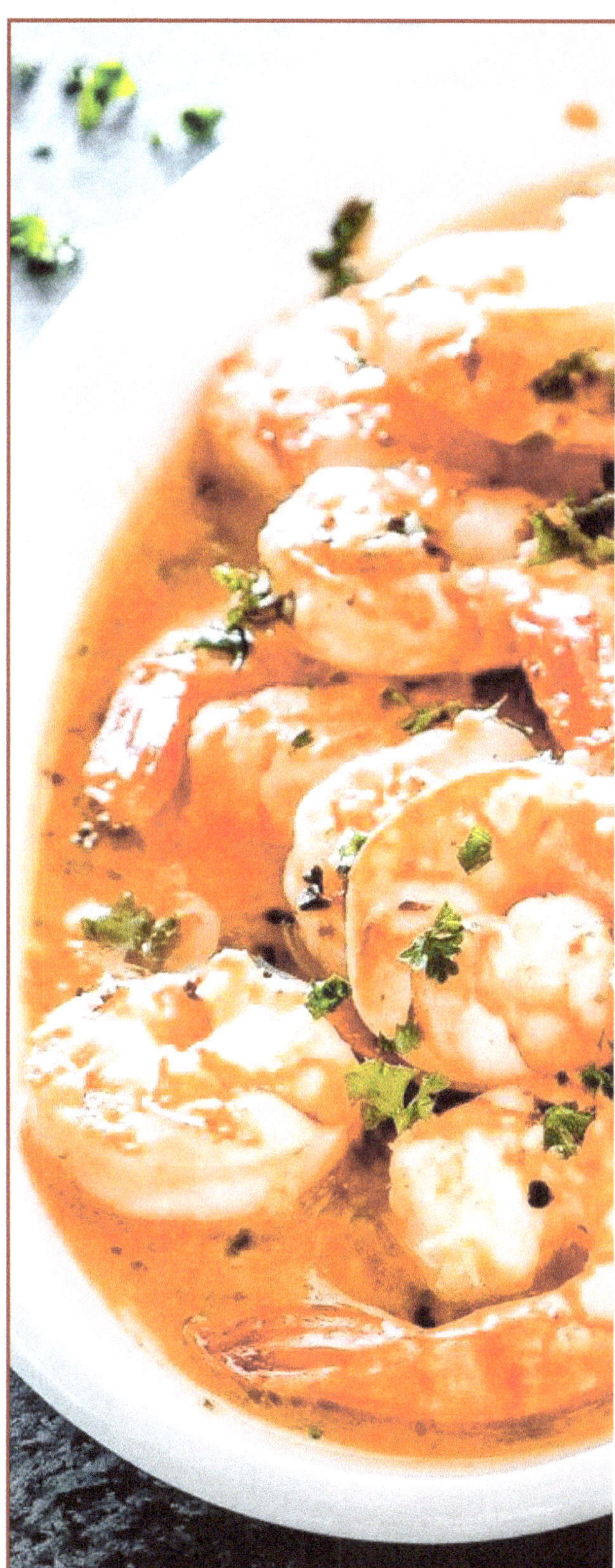

Time of Preparation: 10 minutes
Cooking Time: 10 minutes
Serving Unit: 4 servings

Ingredients:
- 1 pound large shrimp, peeled and deveined
- 4 tablespoons unsalted butter
- 4 cloves garlic, minced
- 1 tablespoon lemon juice
- Salt and pepper to taste
- Optional garnish: chopped fresh parsley, lemon wedges

Procedures:
1. In a large skillet, melt butter over medium heat.
2. Add minced garlic to the skillet and sauté for 1-2 minutes until fragrant.
3. Add shrimp to the skillet and cook for 2-3 minutes on each side until pink and opaque.
4. Drizzle lemon juice over the shrimp and season with salt and pepper to taste.
5. Toss the shrimp in the garlic butter sauce until well coated.
6. Remove from heat and garnish with chopped fresh parsley if desired.
7. Serve hot, with lemon wedges on the side for squeezing over the shrimp.

Cooking Tips:
- Choose large shrimp for this recipe, as they cook quickly and have a nice texture.
- Make sure to devein the shrimp to remove any gritty or sandy residue.
- Be careful not to overcook the shrimp, as they can become tough and rubbery.
- Customize the dish with additional seasonings or herbs, such as red pepper flakes, paprika, or chopped parsley,

- according to your taste preferences.
- Serve the garlic butter shrimp over cooked rice, pasta, or quinoa for a complete meal.

Nutritional Values:
- Calories: Approximately 200 kcal per serving
- Protein: Approximately 20g per serving
- Carbohydrates: Approximately 2g per serving
- Fat: Approximately 12g per serving
- Fiber: Approximately 0g per serving

Health Benefits:
- Shrimp is a low-calorie, high-protein seafood option that's rich in vitamins and minerals, such as vitamin B12, iodine, and selenium, which support thyroid function, metabolism, and immune health.
- Garlic contains sulfur compounds and antioxidants, such as allicin and quercetin, which have antibacterial and anti-inflammatory properties and help boost immune function and protect against chronic diseases.
- Butter provides richness and flavor to the dish while also providing essential fats and calories for energy and satiety.
- Lemon juice adds brightness and acidity to the dish, as well as vitamin C, which supports immune function and collagen production.

Baked Lemon Dill Tilapia

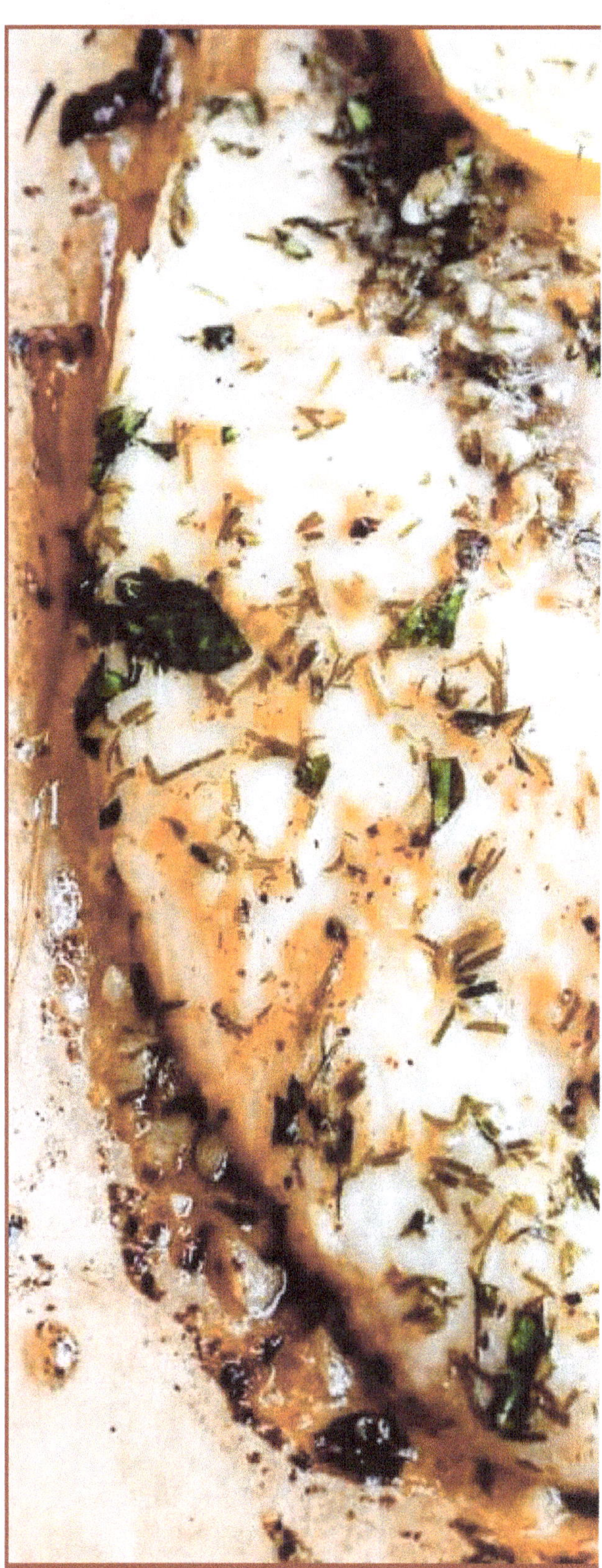

Time of Preparation: 10 minutes
Cooking Time: 15 minutes
Serving Unit: 4 servings

Ingredients:
- 4 tilapia fillets (about 6 ounces each)
- 2 tablespoons olive oil
- 2 tablespoons fresh lemon juice
- 2 teaspoons dried dill weed
- Salt and pepper to taste
- Optional garnish: fresh dill sprigs, lemon wedges

Procedures:
1. Preheat the oven to 400°F (200°C). Line a baking sheet with parchment paper or aluminum foil.
2. Place the tilapia fillets on the prepared baking sheet.
3. In a small bowl, whisk together the olive oil, lemon juice, and dried dill weed.
4. Drizzle the lemon dill mixture over the tilapia fillets, making sure to coat them evenly.
5. Season the tilapia fillets with salt and pepper to taste.
6. Bake in the preheated oven for 12-15 minutes, or until the fish is opaque and flakes easily with a fork.
7. Remove from the oven and let the tilapia rest for a few minutes before serving.
8. Garnish with fresh dill sprigs and lemon wedges if desired.

Cooking Tips:
- Choose tilapia fillets that are firm and have a mild odor, indicating freshness.
- If using frozen tilapia fillets, thaw them completely before baking.
- For extra flavor, you can add minced garlic or grated lemon zest to the lemon dill mixture.

- Be careful not to overcook the tilapia, as it can become dry and rubbery. Check for doneness by gently inserting a fork into the thickest part of the fillet; it should flake easily.
- Serve the baked tilapia with a side of steamed vegetables, rice, or roasted potatoes for a complete and satisfying meal.

Nutritional Values:

- Calories: Approximately 200 kcal per serving
- Protein: Approximately 25g per serving
- Carbohydrates: Approximately 1g per serving
- Fat: Approximately 10g per serving
- Fiber: Approximately 0g per serving

Health Benefits:

- Tilapia is a lean source of protein that's low in calories and saturated fat, making it a healthy option for heart health and weight management.
- Olive oil provides healthy monounsaturated fats, antioxidants, and anti-inflammatory properties, which support heart health, brain function, and overall wellbeing.
- Lemon juice adds brightness and acidity to the dish, as well as vitamin C, which supports immune function and collagen production.
- Dill weed is rich in vitamins, minerals, and antioxidants, such as vitamin A, vitamin C, and flavonoids, which help reduce inflammation, support digestion, and promote overall health and wellbeing.

Seared Tuna Steaks with Sesame Glaze

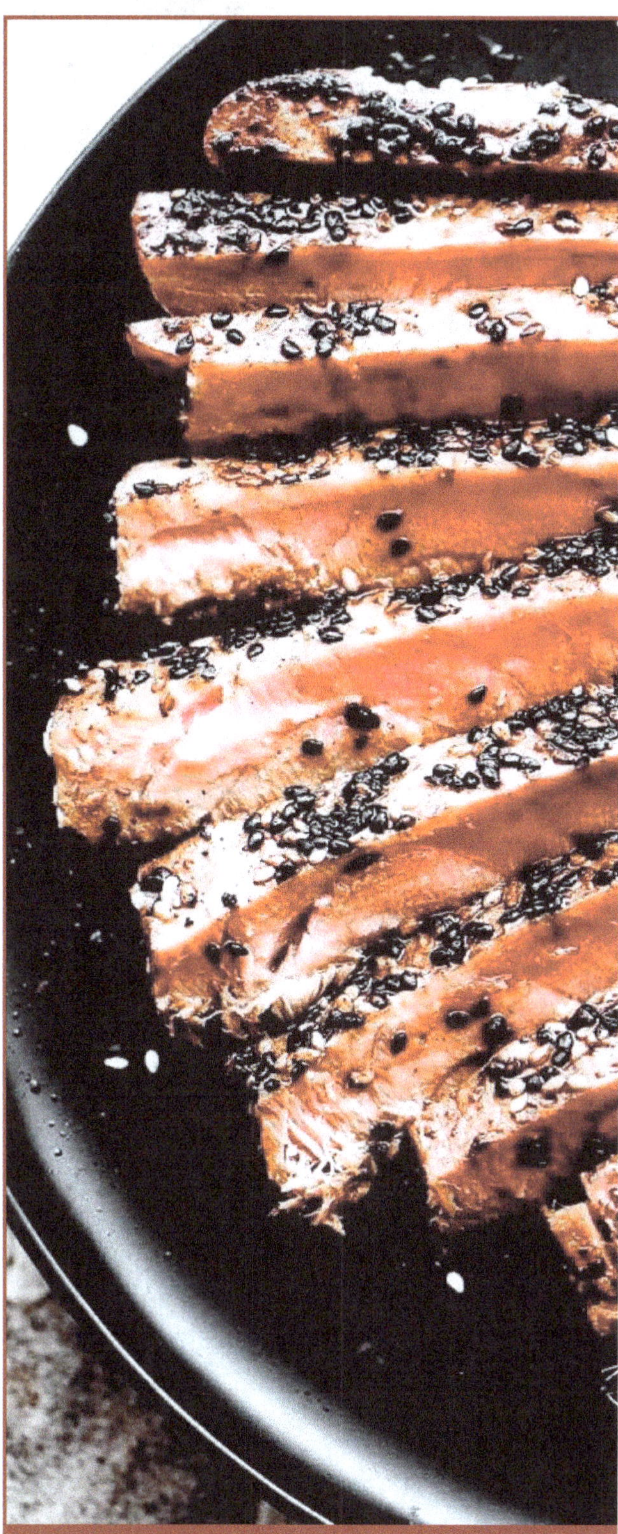

Time of Preparation: 10 minutes
Cooking Time: 5 minutes
Serving Unit: 4 servings

Ingredients:
- 4 tuna steaks (about 6 ounces each)
- 1/4 cup soy sauce
- 2 tablespoons honey
- 1 tablespoon sesame oil
- 1 tablespoon sesame seeds
- Optional garnish: sliced green onions, sesame seeds

Procedures:
1. In a shallow dish or bowl, whisk together the soy sauce, honey, sesame oil, and sesame seeds to make the sesame glaze.
2. Place the tuna steaks in the sesame glaze, turning to coat them evenly. Let them marinate for 5-10 minutes while you preheat the skillet.
3. Heat a skillet or grill pan over medium-high heat. Once hot, add the tuna steaks to the skillet.
4. Sear the tuna steaks for 1-2 minutes on each side, or until the outside is browned and caramelized, but the inside remains pink and tender.
5. Remove the tuna steaks from the skillet and let them rest for a few minutes before slicing.
6. Slice the tuna steaks against the grain into thin slices.
7. Serve hot, garnished with sliced green onions and sesame seeds if desired.

Cooking Tips:
- Choose sushi-grade tuna steaks for the best results, as they are fresh and safe to eat raw or lightly seared.

- Be careful not to overcook the tuna steaks, as they can become dry and tough. Aim for medium-rare to medium doneness for the juiciest and most flavorful results.
- You can adjust the sweetness and saltiness of the sesame glaze to your taste by adding more honey or soy sauce as needed.
- For extra flavor, you can add minced garlic or grated ginger to the sesame glaze.
- Serve the seared tuna steaks with a side of steamed rice, stir-fried vegetables, or a crisp green salad for a complete and satisfying meal.

Nutritional Values:
- Calories: Approximately 250 kcal per serving
- Protein: Approximately 30g per serving
- Carbohydrates: Approximately 10g per serving
- Fat: Approximately 10g per serving
- Fiber: Approximately 1g per serving

Health Benefits:
- Tuna is a lean source of protein that's rich in omega-3 fatty acids, vitamins, and minerals, which support heart health, brain function, and overall wellbeing.
- Soy sauce provides flavor and depth to the dish, as well as protein, vitamins, and minerals, such as iron and potassium, which help regulate blood pressure and support muscle function.
- Honey adds sweetness to the sesame glaze, as well as antioxidants and antibacterial properties, which support immune function and promote wound healing.
- Sesame oil and sesame seeds are rich in healthy fats, antioxidants, and anti-inflammatory compounds, which support heart health, digestion, and skin health.

Mediterranean Style Grilled Swordfish

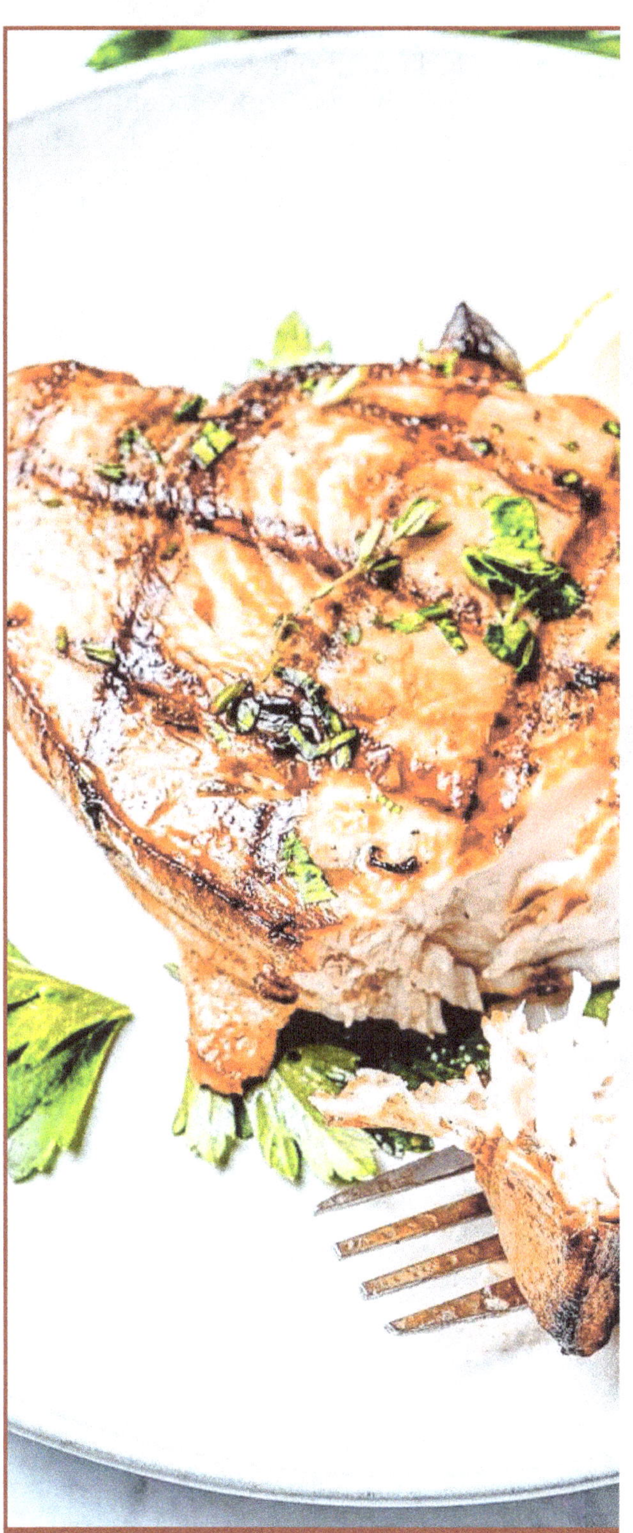

Time of Preparation: 10 minutes
Cooking Time: 10 minutes
Serving Unit: 4 servings

Ingredients:
- 4 swordfish steaks (about 6 ounces each)
- 1/4 cup extra virgin olive oil
- 2 tablespoons lemon juice
- 2 cloves garlic, minced
- 1 tablespoon chopped fresh parsley
- Salt and pepper to taste
- Optional garnish: lemon wedges, chopped fresh parsley

Procedures:
1. In a small bowl, whisk together the olive oil, lemon juice, minced garlic, chopped parsley, salt, and pepper to make the marinade.
2. Place the swordfish steaks in a shallow dish or bowl and pour the marinade over them, turning to coat them evenly. Let them marinate for 10-15 minutes while you preheat the grill.
3. Preheat the grill to medium-high heat. Once hot, lightly oil the grill grates to prevent sticking.
4. Remove the swordfish steaks from the marinade and shake off any excess marinade.
5. Place the swordfish steaks on the preheated grill and cook for 4-5 minutes on each side, or until the fish is opaque and flakes easily with a fork.
6. Remove from the grill and let the swordfish steaks rest for a few minutes before serving.
7. Garnish with lemon wedges and chopped parsley if desired.

Cooking Tips:

- Choose swordfish steaks that are firm, moist, and have a mild odor, indicating freshness.
- Be careful not to overcook the swordfish, as it can become dry and tough. Aim for medium doneness for the juiciest and most flavorful results.
- You can customize the marinade with additional herbs and spices, such as oregano, basil, or red pepper flakes, according to your taste preferences.
- For best results, brush the grill grates with oil before cooking to prevent the fish from sticking.
- Serve the grilled swordfish steaks with a side of roasted vegetables, couscous, or a Greek salad for a complete and satisfying meal.

Nutritional Values:
- Calories: Approximately 300 kcal per serving
- Protein: Approximately 30g per serving
- Carbohydrates: Approximately 2g per serving
- Fat: Approximately 20g per serving
- Fiber: Approximately 0g per serving

Health Benefits:
- Swordfish is a lean source of protein that's rich in omega-3 fatty acids, vitamins, and minerals, which support heart health, brain function, and overall wellbeing.
- Olive oil provides healthy monounsaturated fats, antioxidants, and anti-inflammatory properties, which support heart health, brain function, and overall wellbeing.
- Lemon juice adds brightness and acidity to the dish, as well as vitamin C, which supports immune function and collagen production.
- Garlic and parsley contain sulfur compounds, antioxidants, and anti-inflammatory properties, which support immune function, digestion, and overall health and wellbeing.

Chapter 7: Comforting Poultry Dishes

Chapter 7: Comforting Poultry Dishes

Welcome to Chapter 7, where we explore comforting poultry dishes that are sure to warm your heart and nourish your body. In this chapter, I'll discover a variety of recipes featuring chicken and turkey, from hearty soups and stews to flavorful skillet meals and comforting casseroles.

Poultry is a versatile and lean source of protein that's perfect for diabetes-friendly meals. Whether you're cooking for yourself or feeding your family, you'll find plenty of inspiration in this chapter to create delicious and satisfying poultry dishes that are quick and easy to prepare. Let's dive into the world of comforting poultry dishes and enjoy the comforting goodness they bring to your table!

Herb-Roasted Chicken Thighs

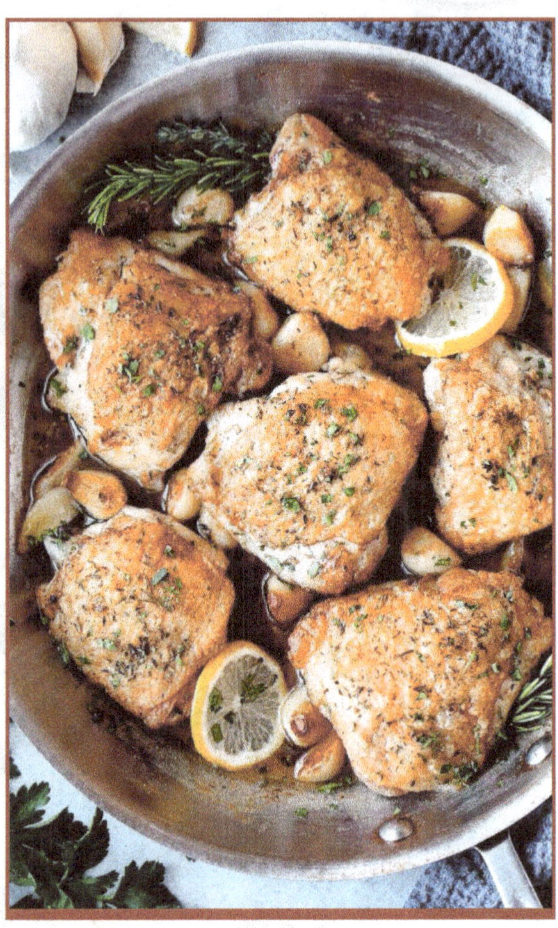

Time of Preparation: 10 minutes
Cooking Time: 25 minutes
Serving Unit: 4 servings

Ingredients:

- 8 bone-in, skin-on chicken thighs
- 2 tablespoons olive oil
- 2 teaspoons dried thyme
- 2 teaspoons dried rosemary
- Salt and pepper to taste
- Optional garnish: fresh thyme or rosemary sprigs
- Lemons

Procedures:

1. Preheat the oven to 425°F (220°C). Line a baking sheet with parchment paper or aluminum foil.
2. Pat the chicken thighs dry with paper towels and place them on the prepared baking sheet.
3. Drizzle the olive oil over the chicken thighs, then sprinkle them with dried thyme, dried rosemary, salt, and pepper.
4. Using your hands, rub the oil and herbs evenly over the chicken thighs to coat them thoroughly.
5. Arrange the chicken thighs in a single layer on the baking sheet, leaving space between them for even cooking.
6. Roast in the preheated oven for 20-25 minutes, or until the chicken thighs are golden brown and cooked through, with an internal temperature of 165°F (74°C).
7. Remove from the oven and let the chicken thighs rest for a few minutes before serving.
8. Garnish with fresh thyme or rosemary sprigs if desired.

Cooking Tips:

- For best results, use bone-in, skin-on chicken thighs, as they are more flavorful and juicy than boneless, skinless ones.
- Make sure to pat the chicken thighs dry with paper towels before seasoning them, as this helps the skin crisp up during roasting.
- Adjust the seasoning according to your taste preferences. You can add other dried herbs such as sage, oregano, or marjoram for additional flavor.
- For extra crispy skin, you can start by searing the chicken thighs in a hot skillet for 2-3 minutes on each side before transferring them to the oven to roast.

- Serve the herb-roasted chicken thighs with your favorite side dishes, such as roasted vegetables, mashed potatoes, or a green salad, for a complete and satisfying meal.

Nutritional Values:

- Calories: Approximately 300 kcal per serving
- Protein: Approximately 25g per serving
- Carbohydrates: Approximately 0g per serving
- Fat: Approximately 22g per serving
- Fiber: Approximately 0g per serving

Health Benefits:

- Chicken thighs are a good source of protein, vitamins, and minerals, such as vitamin B6, niacin, phosphorus, and selenium, which support muscle growth, immune function, and overall wellbeing.
- Olive oil provides healthy monounsaturated fats, antioxidants, and anti-inflammatory properties, which support heart health, brain function, and overall wellbeing.
- Dried thyme and rosemary are rich in antioxidants and anti-inflammatory compounds, such as rosmarinic acid and carnosic acid, which support immune function, digestion, and overall health and wellbeing.

Honey Mustard Glazed Turkey Breast

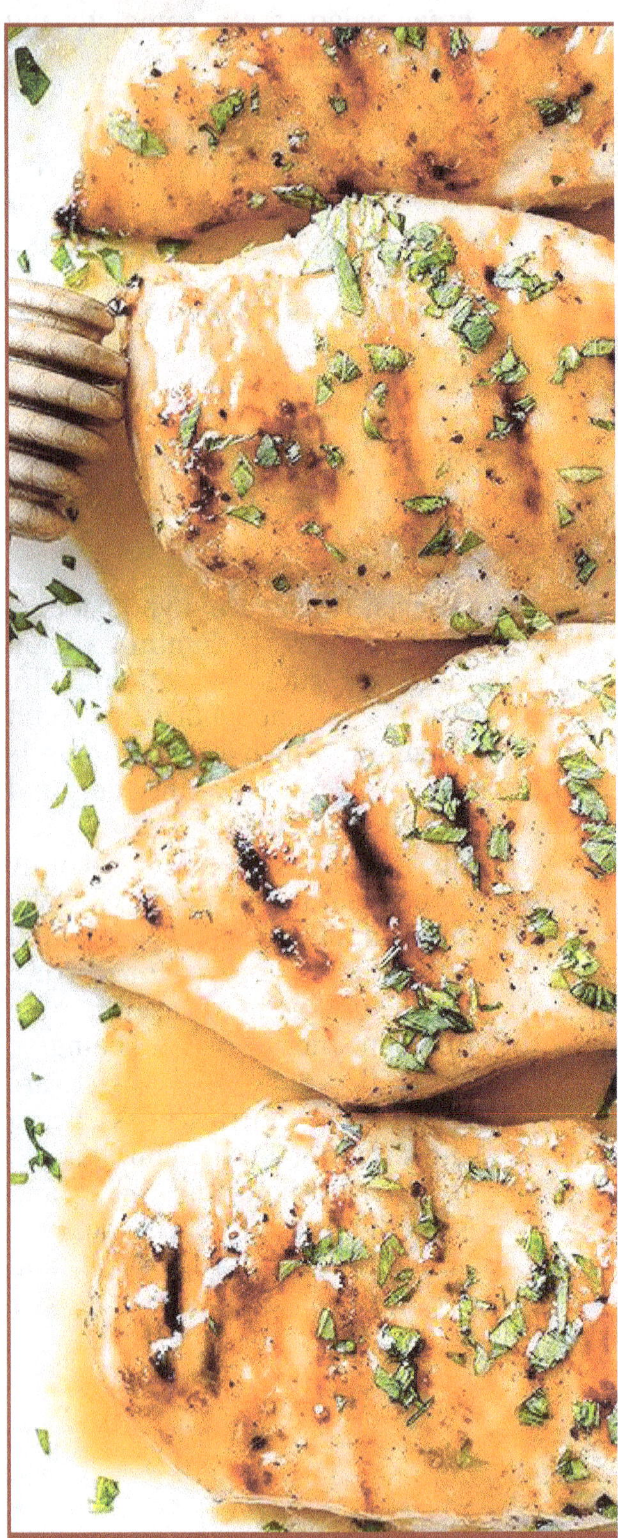

Time of Preparation: 10 minutes
Cooking Time: 20 minutes
Serving Unit: 4 servings

Ingredients:
- 1 turkey breast (about 1 ½ pounds)
- 1/4 cup honey
- 2 tablespoons Dijon mustard
- 1 tablespoon olive oil
- Salt and pepper to taste
- Optional garnish: chopped fresh parsley

Procedures:
1. Preheat the oven to 375°F (190°C). Line a baking dish with parchment paper or aluminum foil.
2. Place the turkey breast in the prepared baking dish.
3. In a small bowl, whisk together the honey, Dijon mustard, olive oil, salt, and pepper to make the glaze.
4. Pour the honey mustard glaze over the turkey breast, spreading it evenly to coat the surface.
5. Roast in the preheated oven for 15-20 minutes, or until the turkey breast is golden brown and cooked through, with an internal temperature of 165°F (74°C).
6. Remove from the oven and let the turkey breast rest for a few minutes before slicing.
7. Garnish with chopped fresh parsley if desired.

Cooking Tips:
- Choose a boneless, skinless turkey breast for this recipe for quicker cooking time and easier slicing.
- Make sure to pat the turkey breast dry with paper towels before adding the glaze, as this helps the glaze adhere better to the surface.

- Adjust the sweetness and tanginess of the glaze according to your taste preferences by adding more or less honey and Dijon mustard.
- For extra flavor, you can add minced garlic or grated ginger to the honey mustard glaze.
- Serve the honey mustard glazed turkey breast with your favorite side dishes, such as roasted vegetables, mashed potatoes, or a leafy green salad, for a complete and satisfying meal.

Nutritional Values:
- Calories: Approximately 250 kcal per serving
- Protein: Approximately 30g per serving
- Carbohydrates: Approximately 10g per serving
- Fat: Approximately 10g per serving
- Fiber: Approximately 0g per serving

Health Benefits:
- Turkey breast is a lean source of protein that's low in fat and calories but high in essential nutrients, such as vitamin B6, niacin, and selenium, which support muscle growth, immune function, and overall wellbeing.
- Honey provides natural sweetness to the dish, as well as antioxidants and antibacterial properties, which support immune function and promote wound healing.
- Dijon mustard adds tanginess and depth to the glaze, as well as vitamins and minerals, such as vitamin C and potassium, which support heart health and digestion.
- Olive oil provides healthy monounsaturated fats, antioxidants, and anti-inflammatory properties, which support heart health, brain function, and overall wellbeing.

Lemon Garlic Chicken Skewers

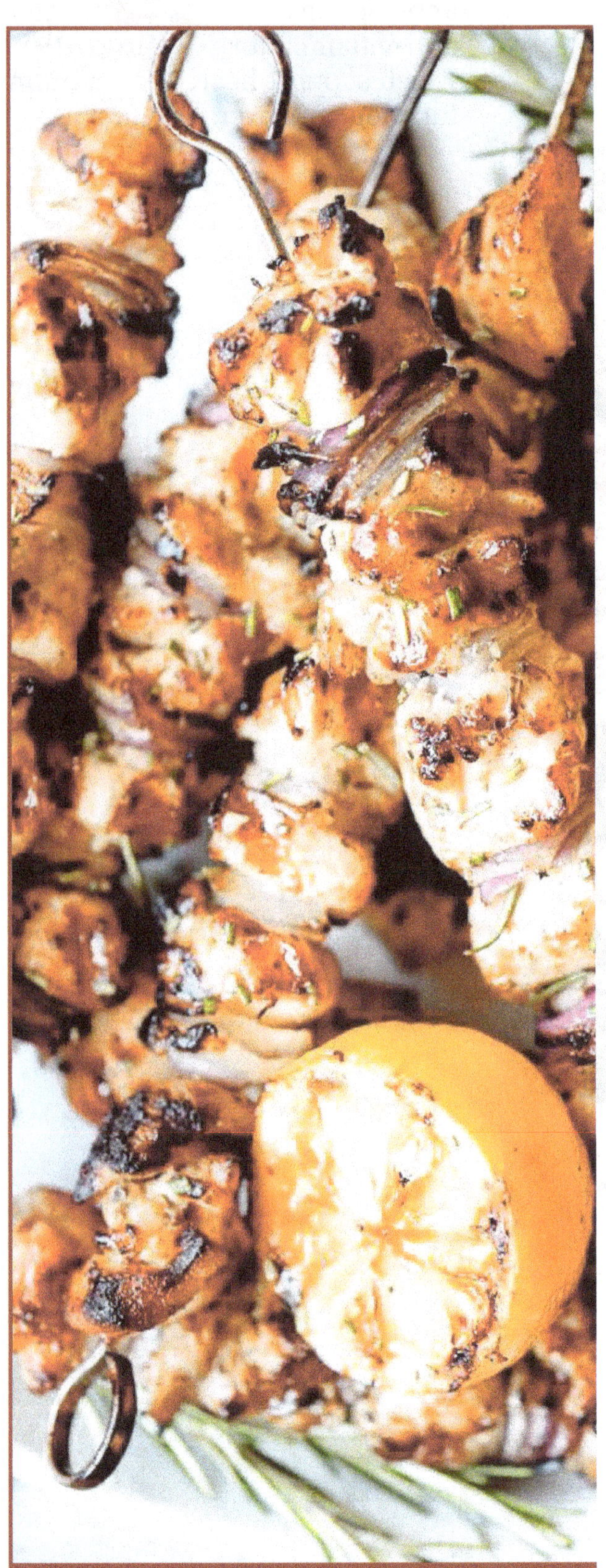

Time of Preparation: 15 minutes
Cooking Time: 10 minutes
Serving Unit: 4 servings

Ingredients:
- 1 pound boneless, skinless chicken breasts, cut into 1-inch cubes
- 2 lemons, juiced and zested
- 4 cloves garlic, minced
- 2 tablespoons olive oil
- Salt and pepper to taste

Procedures:
1. In a mixing bowl, combine the lemon juice, lemon zest, minced garlic, olive oil, salt, and pepper. Stir until well combined to create the marinade.
2. Add the chicken cubes to the marinade and toss to coat evenly. Cover the bowl and let the chicken marinate in the refrigerator for at least 15 minutes, or up to 1 hour, to allow the flavors to meld together.
3. While the chicken is marinating, preheat your grill or grill pan over medium-high heat.
4. Thread the marinated chicken cubes onto skewers, leaving a small space between each piece to ensure even cooking.
5. Once the grill is hot, place the chicken skewers on the grill and cook for 4-5 minutes on each side, or until the chicken is cooked through and golden brown, with grill marks.
6. Remove the chicken skewers from the grill and transfer them to a serving platter.
7. Garnish the Lemon Garlic Chicken Skewers with additional lemon slices and chopped fresh herbs, if desired.
8. Serve immediately, and enjoy!

Cooking Tips:

- Soak wooden skewers in water for at least 30 minutes before threading the chicken onto them to prevent them from burning on the grill.
- Use metal skewers for a quicker cooking time and easy cleanup.
- Customize the marinade with additional herbs and spices, such as chopped rosemary, thyme, or red pepper flakes, for added flavor and heat.
- Serve the chicken skewers with a side of rice, quinoa, or grilled vegetables for a complete and satisfying meal.

Nutritional Values:
- Calories: Approximately 200 kcal per serving (2 skewers)
- Protein: Approximately 25g per serving
- Carbohydrates: Approximately 4g per serving
- Fat: Approximately 10g per serving
- Fiber: Approximately 1g per serving
-

Health Benefits:
- Chicken is a lean source of protein that's low in calories and saturated fat but high in essential nutrients, including vitamins B6 and B12, which support energy metabolism and immune function.
- Lemons are rich in vitamin C, antioxidants, and soluble fiber, which support immune health, skin health, and digestion, and may help reduce the risk of chronic diseases.
- Garlic contains sulfur compounds with potential health benefits, including anti-inflammatory and antimicrobial properties, which may help boost immune function and reduce the risk of infections.
- Olive oil is rich in heart-healthy monounsaturated fats and antioxidants, which may help reduce inflammation, lower cholesterol levels, and protect against heart disease and stroke.

BBQ Chicken Skewers

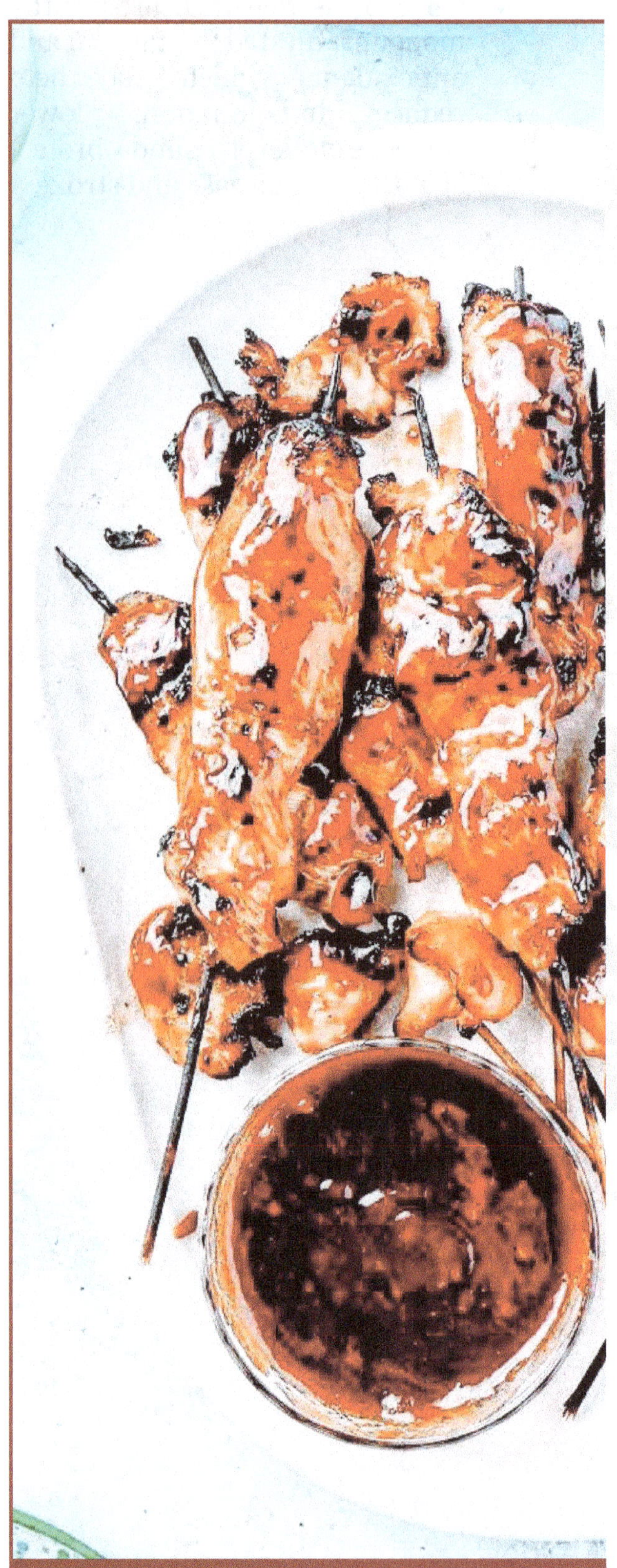

Time of Preparation: 15 minutes
Cooking Time: 10 minutes
Serving Unit: 4 servings

Ingredients:

- 1 pound boneless, skinless chicken breasts, cut into 1-inch cubes
- 1/2 cup BBQ sauce
- 2 tablespoons olive oil
- Salt and pepper to taste
- Optional garnish: chopped fresh cilantro or green onions

Procedures:

1. Preheat the grill to medium-high heat.
2. In a mixing bowl, combine the chicken cubes, BBQ sauce, olive oil, salt, and pepper. Toss until the chicken is evenly coated with the BBQ sauce mixture.
3. Thread the chicken cubes onto skewers, leaving a little space between each piece.
4. Once the grill is hot, lightly oil the grill grates to prevent sticking.
5. Place the chicken skewers on the grill and cook for 4-5 minutes on each side, or until the chicken is cooked through and has grill marks.
6. Remove the chicken skewers from the grill and transfer them to a serving platter.
7. Garnish with chopped fresh cilantro or green onions if desired.

Cooking Tips:

- If using wooden skewers, soak them in water for at least 30 minutes before threading the chicken onto them. This prevents them from burning on the grill.
- Cut the chicken into evenly sized cubes to ensure even cooking.
- You can use your favorite BBQ sauce for this recipe, whether

store-bought or homemade. Choose a sauce that complements the flavor of the chicken.

- Baste the chicken skewers with extra BBQ sauce while grilling for extra flavor and moisture.
- Serve the BBQ chicken skewers with your favorite side dishes, such as coleslaw, potato salad, or grilled vegetables, for a complete and satisfying meal.

Nutritional Values:
- Calories: Approximately 250 kcal per serving
- Protein: Approximately 25g per serving
- Carbohydrates: Approximately 15g per serving
- Fat: Approximately 10g per serving
- Fiber: Approximately 1g per serving

Health Benefits:
- Chicken breast is a lean source of protein that's low in fat and calories but high in essential nutrients, such as vitamin B6, niacin, and selenium, which support muscle growth, immune function, and overall wellbeing.
- BBQ sauce provides flavor and moisture to the chicken skewers, as well as antioxidants and anti-inflammatory properties, which support heart health and digestion.
- Olive oil adds healthy monounsaturated fats to the dish, which support heart health and brain function.
- Fresh cilantro or green onions add freshness and color to the dish, as well as vitamins and minerals, such as vitamin K and folate, which support immune function and bone health.

Chapter 8: Wholesome Vegetarian Delights

Chapter 8: Wholesome Vegetarian Delights

Welcome to Chapter 8 where we celebrate the goodness of vegetarian cuisine. In this chapter, we explore a variety of wholesome and flavorful vegetarian dishes that are not only delicious but also perfect for managing blood sugar levels and promoting overall health.

Vegetarian meals are rich in fiber, vitamins, and minerals, making them ideal choices for individuals with type 2 diabetes. From vibrant salads and hearty soups to satisfying mains and nutritious sides, you'll find plenty of inspiration in this chapter to create delicious and nourishing vegetarian meals that everyone will love.

Whether you're a dedicated vegetarian or simply looking to incorporate more plant-based foods into your diet, these recipes will show you just how delicious and satisfying vegetarian cooking can be. Let's embark on a culinary journey and discover the joy of wholesome vegetarian delights together!

Mushroom and Spinach Quesadillas

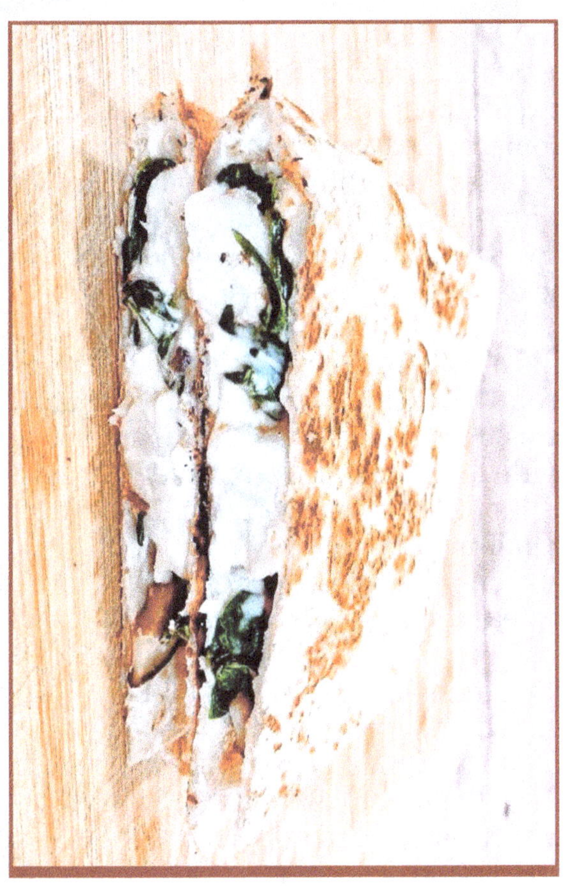

Time of Preparation: **15** minutes
Cooking Time: 10 minutes
Serving Unit: 4 servings

Ingredients:
- 8 whole wheat tortillas
- 2 cups sliced mushrooms
- 2 cups fresh spinach leaves
- 1 cup shredded cheese (such as Monterey Jack or cheddar)
- 2 tablespoons olive oil
- Salt and pepper to taste
- Optional garnish: salsa, guacamole, sour cream

Procedures:

1. In a large skillet, heat 1 tablespoon of olive oil over medium heat.

2. Add the sliced mushrooms to the skillet and sauté for 5-6 minutes, or until they are golden brown and tender. Season with salt and pepper to taste. Remove the mushrooms from the skillet and set aside.

3. In the same skillet, add the remaining 1 tablespoon of olive oil. Add the fresh spinach leaves and sauté for 2-3 minutes, or until they are wilted. Season with salt and pepper to taste. Remove the spinach from the skillet and set aside.

4. Place one tortilla in the skillet and sprinkle half of it with shredded cheese. Top the cheese with a layer of sautéed mushrooms and spinach, then sprinkle with additional cheese. Fold the other half of the tortilla over the filling to form a half-moon shape.

5. Cook the quesadilla for 2-3 minutes on each side, or until it is golden brown and the cheese is melted. Repeat with the remaining tortillas and filling ingredients.

6. Once all the quesadillas are cooked, slice them into wedges and serve hot with salsa, guacamole, and sour cream on the side if desired.

Cooking Tips:

- Use whole wheat tortillas for added fiber and nutrients.
- Feel free to customize the filling with your favorite vegetables or additional ingredients such as bell peppers, onions, or black beans.
- You can use any type of cheese you prefer for this recipe, but I recommend using a cheese that melts well, such as Monterey Jack or cheddar.
- Make sure not to overfill the quesadillas, as this can make them difficult to flip and may cause the filling to spill out.
- Serve the quesadillas with a variety of toppings and dipping sauces for extra flavor and enjoyment.

Nutritional Values:

- Calories: Approximately 300 kcal per serving (1 quesadilla)
- Protein: Approximately 10g per serving
- Carbohydrates: Approximately 30g per serving
- Fat: Approximately 15g per serving
- Fiber: Approximately 5g per serving

Health Benefits:

- Mushrooms are low in calories and carbohydrates but rich in vitamins, minerals, and antioxidants, which support immune function, digestion, and overall health and wellbeing.
- Spinach is a nutrient-dense leafy green vegetable that's rich in vitamins, minerals, and antioxidants, such as vitamin A, vitamin C, iron, and folate, which support immune function, bone health, and eye health.
- Olive oil provides healthy monounsaturated fats, antioxidants, and anti-inflammatory properties, which support heart health, brain function, and overall wellbeing.
- Whole wheat tortillas provide fiber, vitamins, and minerals, which support digestive health, blood sugar control, and weight management.

RACHEAL BLAKE

Baked Cod with Herbs

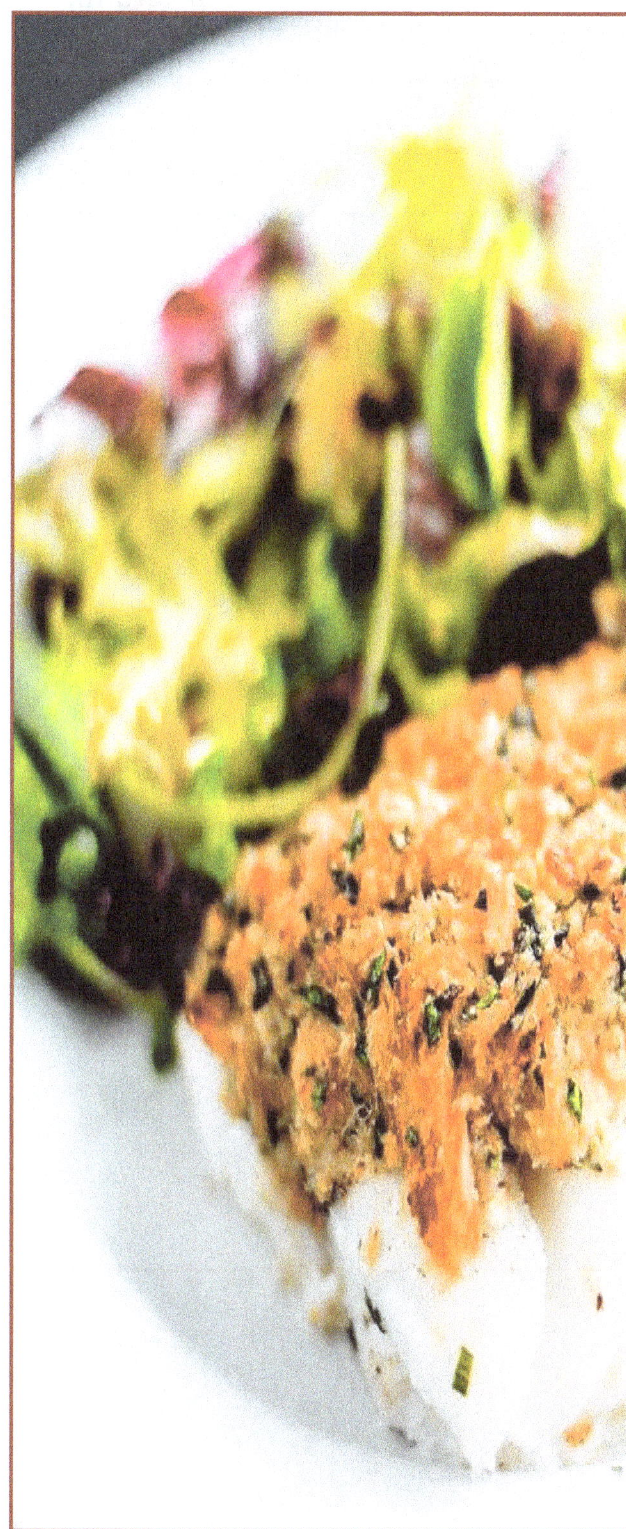

Cooking Time: 15 minutes
Serving Unit: 4 servings

Ingredients:
- 4 cod filets (about 6 ounces each)
- 2 tablespoons olive oil
- 2 cloves garlic, minced
- 2 tablespoons chopped fresh herbs (such as parsley, dill, or thyme)
- Salt and pepper to taste
- Optional: lemon wedges for serving

Procedures:
1. Preheat the oven to 400°F (200°C). Line a baking sheet with parchment paper or aluminum foil for easy cleanup.
2. Place the cod fillets on the prepared baking sheet, leaving some space between them.
3. Drizzle the olive oil over the cod fillets, then sprinkle the minced garlic and chopped fresh herbs on top.
4. Season the cod fillets with salt and pepper to taste, ensuring even seasoning on both sides.
5. Bake the cod fillets in the preheated oven for 12-15 minutes, or until they are opaque and flake easily with a fork.
6. Once the cod fillets are cooked through, remove them from the oven and transfer them to serving plates.
7. Optional: Serve the Baked Cod with Herbs with lemon wedges on the side for added freshness and flavor.
8. Serve immediately, and enjoy!

Cooking Tips:
- Choose fresh, high-quality cod fillets for the best flavor and texture in the dish.
- Use a mixture of your favorite fresh herbs, such as parsley, dill, thyme, or cilantro, for added flavor and aroma.

Time of Preparation: 10 minutes

- Adjust the amount of garlic and herbs according to your taste preferences, or omit them altogether for a simpler preparation.
- For a crispier texture, you can broil the cod fillets for 1-2 minutes at the end of the cooking time, but be careful not to overcook them.
- Serve the Baked Cod with Herbs with your favorite side dishes, such as roasted vegetables, steamed rice, or a fresh salad, for a complete and balanced meal.

Nutritional Values:
- Calories: Approximately 200 kcal per serving
- Protein: Approximately 25g per serving
- Carbohydrates: Approximately 1g per serving
- Fat: Approximately 10g per serving
- Fiber: Approximately 0g per serving

Health Benefits:
- Cod is a lean source of protein and is rich in vitamins and minerals, including vitamin B12, vitamin D, and selenium, which support muscle growth, bone health, and immune function.
- Olive oil is rich in heart-healthy monounsaturated fats and antioxidants, including oleic acid and polyphenols, which may help reduce inflammation, lower cholesterol levels, and protect against heart disease and stroke.
- Garlic is known for its antibacterial and anti-inflammatory properties, and contains vitamins and minerals, including vitamin C, vitamin B6, and manganese, which support immune function, heart health, and bone health.
- Fresh herbs add flavor, aroma, and nutrients to the dish, and are rich in vitamins, minerals, and antioxidants, including vitamin K, vitamin C, and flavonoids, which support overall health and well-being.

Stir-Fried Broccoli and Tofu

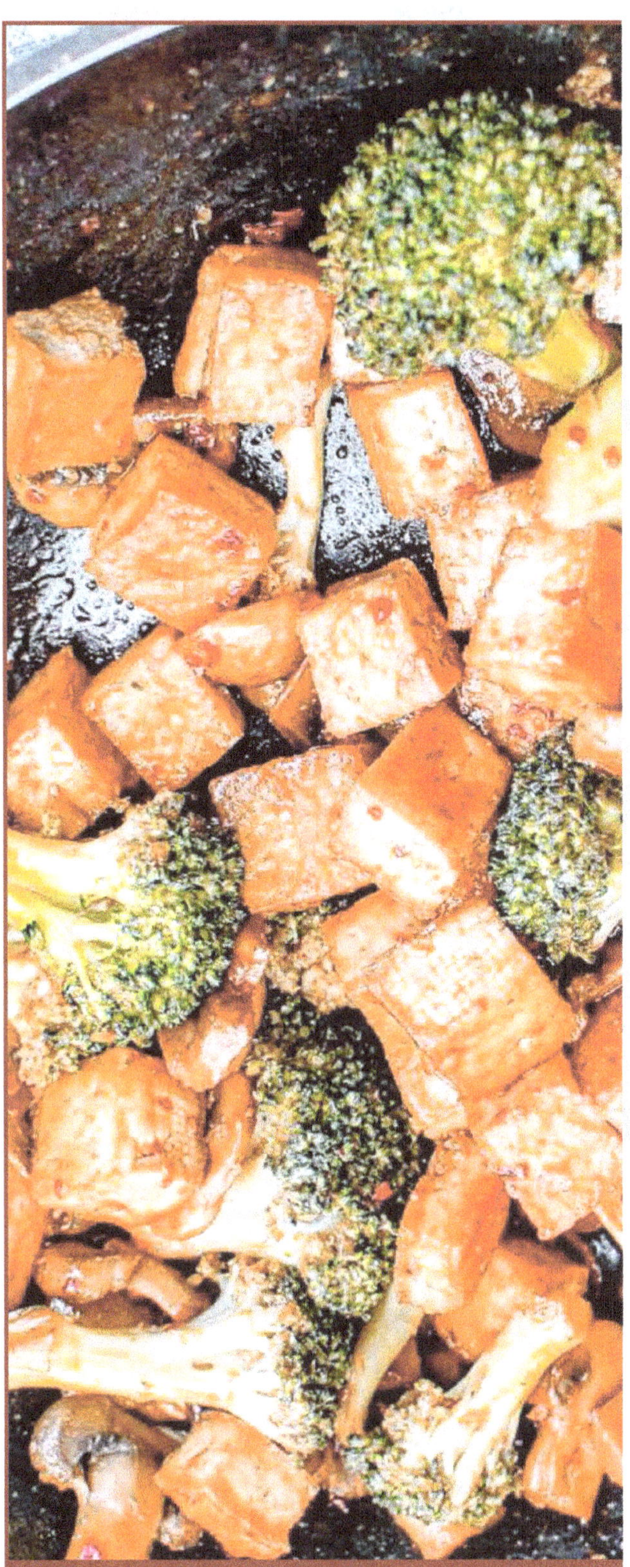

Time of Preparation: 10 minutes
Cooking Time: 15 minutes
Serving Unit: 2 servings

Ingredients:
- 1 block (14 ounces) firm tofu, drained and pressed
- 2 cups broccoli florets
- 2 tablespoons soy sauce (or tamari for a gluten-free option)
- 1 tablespoon sesame oil (or vegetable oil)
- 2 cloves garlic, minced
- Optional: sesame seeds or sliced green onions for garnish

Procedures:
1. Cut the pressed tofu into bite-sized cubes.
2. Heat sesame oil in a large skillet or wok over medium-high heat.
3. Add the minced garlic to the skillet and sauté for 1 minute, until fragrant.
4. Add the tofu cubes to the skillet and cook for 5-6 minutes, stirring occasionally, until golden brown and crispy on all sides.
5. Add the broccoli florets to the skillet and cook for an additional 3-4 minutes, until tender-crisp.
6. Drizzle soy sauce over the tofu and broccoli in the skillet and toss to coat evenly.
7. Cook for another 1-2 minutes, until the sauce is heated through and the flavors are well combined.
8. Remove the skillet from the heat and transfer the Stir-Fried Broccoli and Tofu to serving plates.
9. Garnish with sesame seeds or sliced green onions, if desired.
10. Serve immediately, and enjoy!

Cooking Tips:
- Pressing the tofu before cooking helps remove excess moisture,

- allowing it to crisp up better in the skillet.
- Use firm or extra-firm tofu for stir-frying, as it holds its shape better and has a denser texture.
- Customize the stir-fry with additional vegetables, such as bell peppers, carrots, or snap peas, for added flavor, color, and nutrition.
- For added heat and flavor, you can add a dash of sriracha or chili flakes to the stir-fry sauce.
- Serve the Stir-Fried Broccoli and Tofu over cooked rice or noodles for a complete and satisfying meal.

Nutritional Values:
- Calories: Approximately 250 kcal per serving
- Protein: Approximately 18g per serving
- Carbohydrates: Approximately 12g per serving
- Fat: Approximately 15g per serving
- Fiber: Approximately 4g per serving

Health Benefits:
- Tofu is a versatile plant-based protein that's low in calories and cholesterol but high in protein, calcium, and iron, making it a nutritious alternative to meat.
- Broccoli is a cruciferous vegetable that's rich in vitamins, minerals, and antioxidants, including vitamin C, vitamin K, and folate, which support immune function, bone health, and cardiovascular health.
- Soy sauce (or tamari) adds flavor and depth to the stir-fry, but choose low-sodium options to reduce sodium intake.
- Sesame oil provides a nutty aroma and flavor to the dish, as well as heart-healthy monounsaturated fats and antioxidants, which may help reduce inflammation and cholesterol levels.
- This dish is low in calories and carbohydrates but high in protein, fiber, and essential nutrients, making it a nutritious and satisfying option for individuals looking to maintain a healthy weight or improve their overall diet.

Spicy Black Bean Tacos

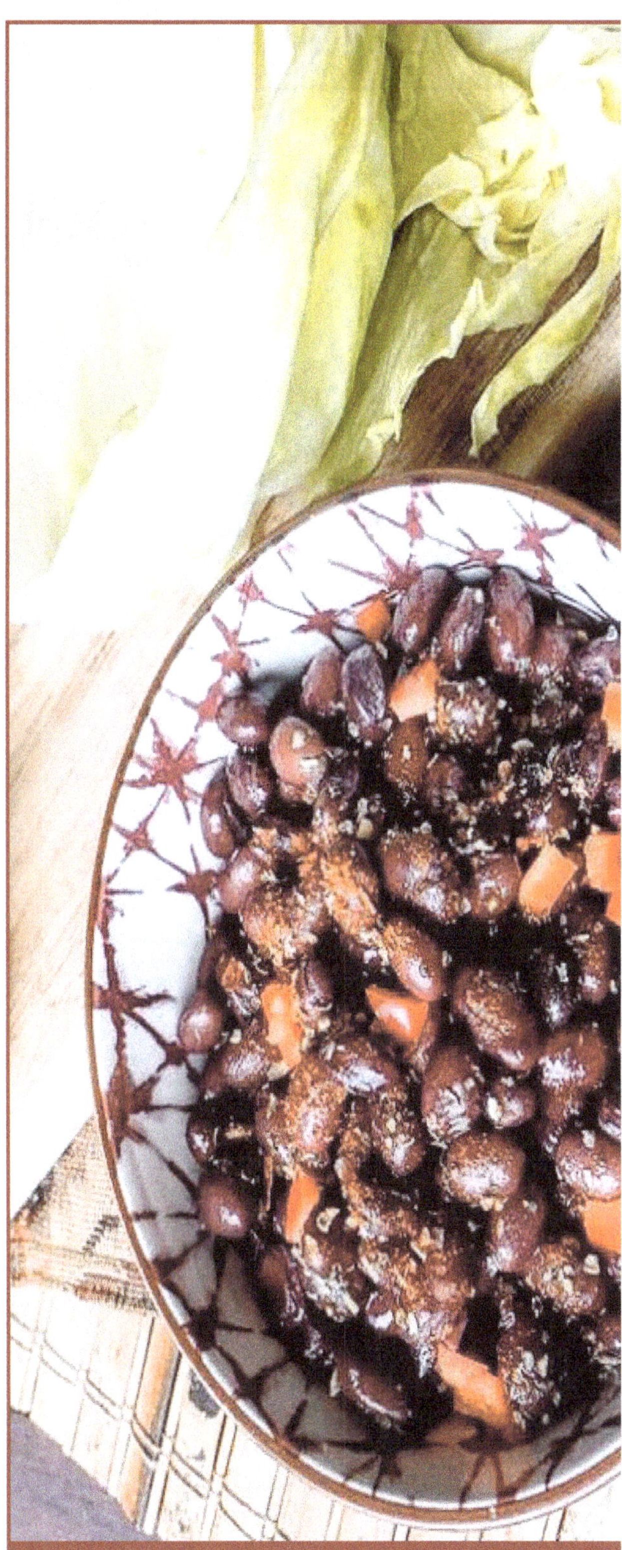

Time of Preparation: 10 minutes
Cooking Time: 15 minutes
Serving Unit: 4 servings (2 tacos per serving)

Ingredients:

- 1 can (15 ounces) black beans, drained and rinsed
- 1 tablespoon taco seasoning (store-bought or homemade)
- 8 small corn tortillas
- 1 cup shredded lettuce
- 1/2 cup diced tomatoes
- Optional toppings: sliced avocado, chopped cilantro, salsa, lime wedges

Procedures:

1. In a medium saucepan, heat the drained and rinsed black beans over medium heat.

2. Add the taco seasoning to the black beans and stir to combine. Cook for 5-7 minutes, stirring occasionally, until the beans are heated through and the seasoning is well incorporated.

3. While the black beans are cooking, warm the corn tortillas in a dry skillet over medium heat for 1-2 minutes on each side, until soft and pliable.

4. Once the black beans are heated through, remove them from the heat and set aside.

5. To assemble the tacos, place a spoonful of the seasoned black beans onto each warm corn tortilla.

6. Top the black beans with shredded lettuce and diced tomatoes.

7. Add any optional toppings, such as sliced avocado, chopped cilantro, salsa, or lime wedges, according to your preference.

8. Serve the Spicy Black Bean Tacos immediately, and enjoy!

Cooking Tips:

- Customize the taco seasoning to your taste preferences by adjusting the amount of chili powder, cumin, paprika, garlic powder, and salt.
- Choose low-sodium black beans and taco seasoning for a healthier option.
- Warm the corn tortillas before assembling the tacos to make them more pliable and easier to fold without cracking.
- Add a squeeze of fresh lime juice over the tacos for added flavor and acidity.
- Serve the tacos with a side of Mexican rice, refried beans, or a simple salad for a complete and satisfying meal.

Nutritional Values:

- Calories: Approximately 200 kcal per serving (2 tacos)
- Protein: Approximately 8g per serving
- Carbohydrates: Approximately 35g per serving
- Fat: Approximately 3g per serving
- Fiber: Approximately 8g per serving

Health Benefits:

- Black beans are a good source of plant-based protein, fiber, vitamins, and minerals, including folate, magnesium, and iron, which support digestive health, heart health, and blood sugar control, and may help reduce the risk of chronic diseases.
- Corn tortillas are gluten-free and lower in calories and carbohydrates than flour tortillas, making them a suitable option for individuals with gluten sensitivities or those looking to reduce their carb intake.
- Lettuce and tomatoes are low in calories and high in fiber, vitamins, and antioxidants, including vitamin C and vitamin A, which support immune function, eye health, and skin health.
- Avocado is rich in heart-healthy monounsaturated fats, fiber, vitamins, and minerals, including potassium and vitamin E, which support heart health, cholesterol levels, and skin health.

Lentil and Vegetable Curry

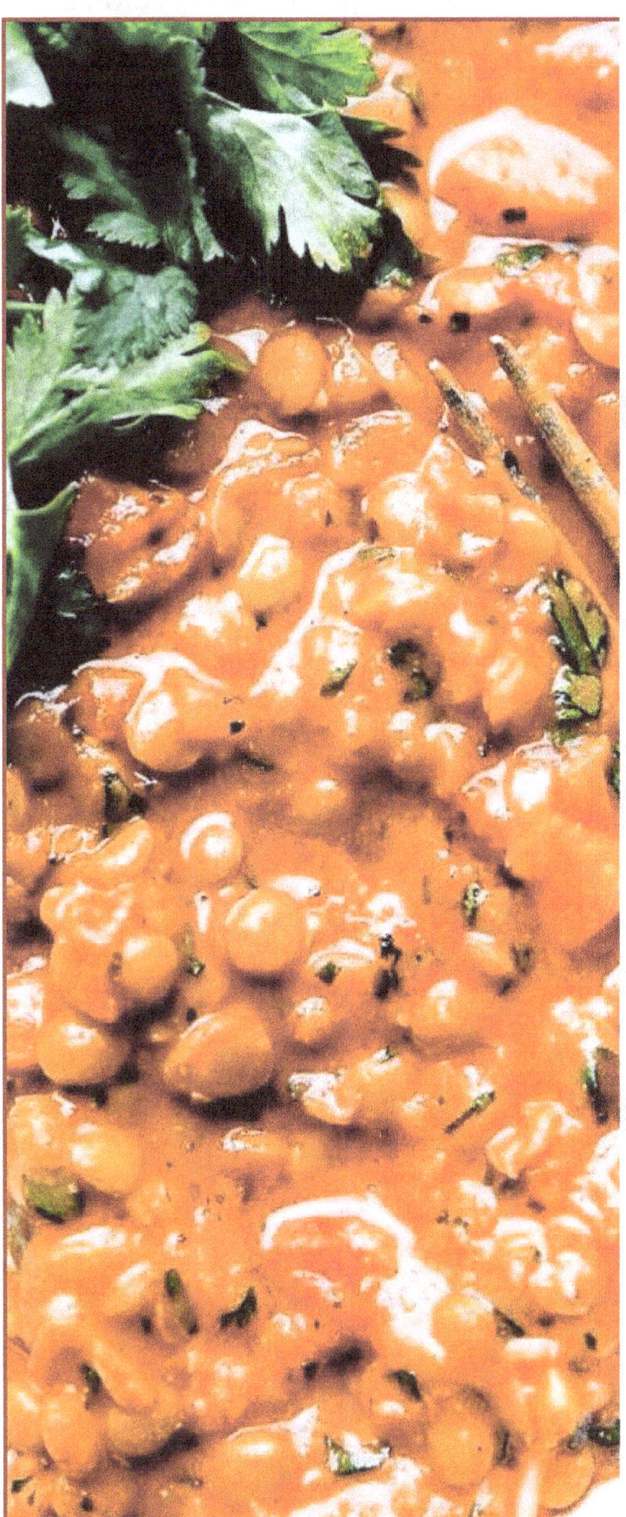

Time of Preparation: 10 minutes
Cooking Time: 20 minutes
Serving Unit: 4 servings

Ingredients:
- 1 cup dried lentils
- 2 cups chopped mixed vegetables (such as bell peppers, carrots, cauliflower, and peas)
- 1 can (14 oz) coconut milk
- 2 tablespoons curry powder
- 2 tablespoons olive oil
- Salt and pepper to taste
- Optional garnish: chopped fresh cilantro, lime wedges

Procedures:
1. Rinse the dried lentils under cold water and drain them. Set aside.
2. In a large skillet or saucepan, heat the olive oil over medium heat.
3. Add the chopped mixed vegetables to the skillet and sauté for 5-6 minutes, or until they are slightly softened.
4. Stir in the curry powder and cook for an additional 1-2 minutes, until fragrant.
5. Add the rinsed lentils and coconut milk to the skillet, stirring to combine.
6. Bring the mixture to a simmer, then reduce the heat to low and cover the skillet. Let the curry simmer for 15-20 minutes, or until the lentils and vegetables are tender and cooked through.
7. Season the curry with salt and pepper to taste, adjusting the seasoning as needed.
8. Serve the lentil and vegetable curry hot, garnished with chopped fresh cilantro and lime wedges if desired.

Cooking Tips:
- Use any combination of your favorite vegetables for this curry. Bell peppers, carrots, cauliflower, and peas work well, but feel free to customize it to your taste.

- Adjust the spice level of the curry by adding more or less curry powder according to your preference.
- For extra creaminess, you can use full-fat coconut milk instead of light coconut milk.
- Serve the curry with cooked rice or naan bread for a complete and satisfying meal.
- Store any leftovers in an airtight container in the refrigerator for up to 3 days. Reheat gently on the stovetop or in the microwave before serving.

Nutritional Values:
- Calories: Approximately 300 kcal per serving
- Protein: Approximately 10g per serving
- Carbohydrates: Approximately 30g per serving
- Fat: Approximately 15g per serving
- Fiber: Approximately 10g per serving

Health Benefits:
- Lentils are a rich source of plant-based protein, fiber, vitamins, and minerals, which support digestive health, blood sugar control, and heart health.
- Mixed vegetables provide a variety of vitamins, minerals, and antioxidants, such as vitamin C, vitamin A, and potassium, which support immune function, eye health, and overall wellbeing.
- Coconut milk adds creaminess and richness to the curry, as well as healthy fats and medium-chain triglycerides, which support heart health and brain function.
- Olive oil provides healthy monounsaturated fats, antioxidants, and anti-inflammatory properties, which support heart health, brain function, and overall wellbeing.

Grilled Portobello Mushroom Burgers

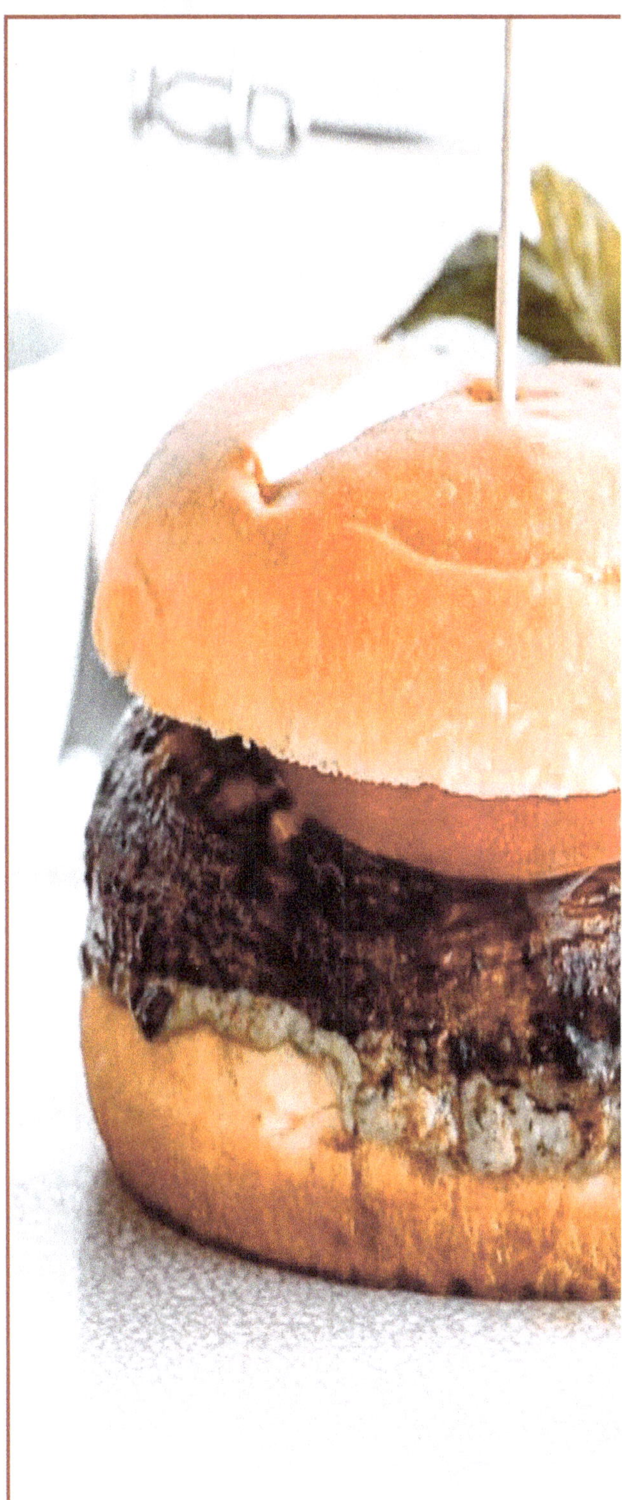

Time of Preparation: 10 minutes
Cooking Time: 10 minutes
Serving Unit: 4 servings

Ingredients:
- 4 large portobello mushroom caps
- 4 whole wheat burger buns
- 1/2 cup balsamic vinegar
- 2 tablespoons olive oil
- Salt and pepper to taste
- Optional toppings: sliced tomatoes, lettuce, avocado, onions, cheese

Procedures:
1. Preheat the grill to medium-high heat.
2. In a small bowl, whisk together the balsamic vinegar and olive oil to make the marinade.
3. Clean the portobello mushroom caps and remove the stems. Place them in a shallow dish or bowl and pour the marinade over them, turning to coat them evenly. Let them marinate for 5-10 minutes while the grill heats up.
4. Once the grill is hot, lightly oil the grill grates to prevent sticking.
5. Place the portobello mushroom caps on the grill, gill side down, and cook for 4-5 minutes on each side, or until they are tender and have grill marks.
6. While the mushrooms are grilling, toast the burger buns on the grill for 1-2 minutes, until lightly browned.
7. Remove the portobello mushroom caps and burger buns from the grill.
8. Assemble the burgers by placing a grilled portobello mushroom cap on each burger bun. Add your favorite toppings, such as sliced tomatoes, lettuce, avocado, onions, and cheese.
9. Serve the grilled portobello mushroom burgers hot, with your

favorite side dishes, such as sweet potato fries or a green salad.

Cooking Tips:
- Choose large portobello mushroom caps that are firm and clean, with no signs of bruising or discoloration.
- You can customize the marinade by adding garlic, herbs, or spices to suit your taste preferences.
- Be careful not to overcook the portobello mushroom caps, as they can become mushy. Aim for a tender texture with slightly charred grill marks.
- Feel free to add additional toppings and condiments to your burgers, such as mustard, ketchup, or mayonnaise.
- Serve the grilled portobello mushroom burgers on whole wheat burger buns for added fiber and nutrients.

Nutritional Values:
- Calories: Approximately 200 kcal per serving (1 burger)
- Protein: Approximately 5g per serving
- Carbohydrates: Approximately 30g per serving
- Fat: Approximately 8g per serving
- Fiber: Approximately 5g per serving

Health Benefits:
- Portobello mushrooms are low in calories and carbohydrates but rich in vitamins, minerals, and antioxidants, such as vitamin D, selenium, and potassium, which support immune function, bone health, and overall wellbeing.
- Balsamic vinegar adds tanginess and flavor to the mushrooms, as well as antioxidants and anti-inflammatory properties, which support heart health and digestion.
- Olive oil provides healthy monounsaturated fats, antioxidants, and anti-inflammatory properties, which support heart health, brain function, and overall wellbeing.
- Whole wheat burger buns provide fiber, vitamins, and minerals, which support digestive health, blood sugar control, and weight management.

Tomato Basil Bruschetta

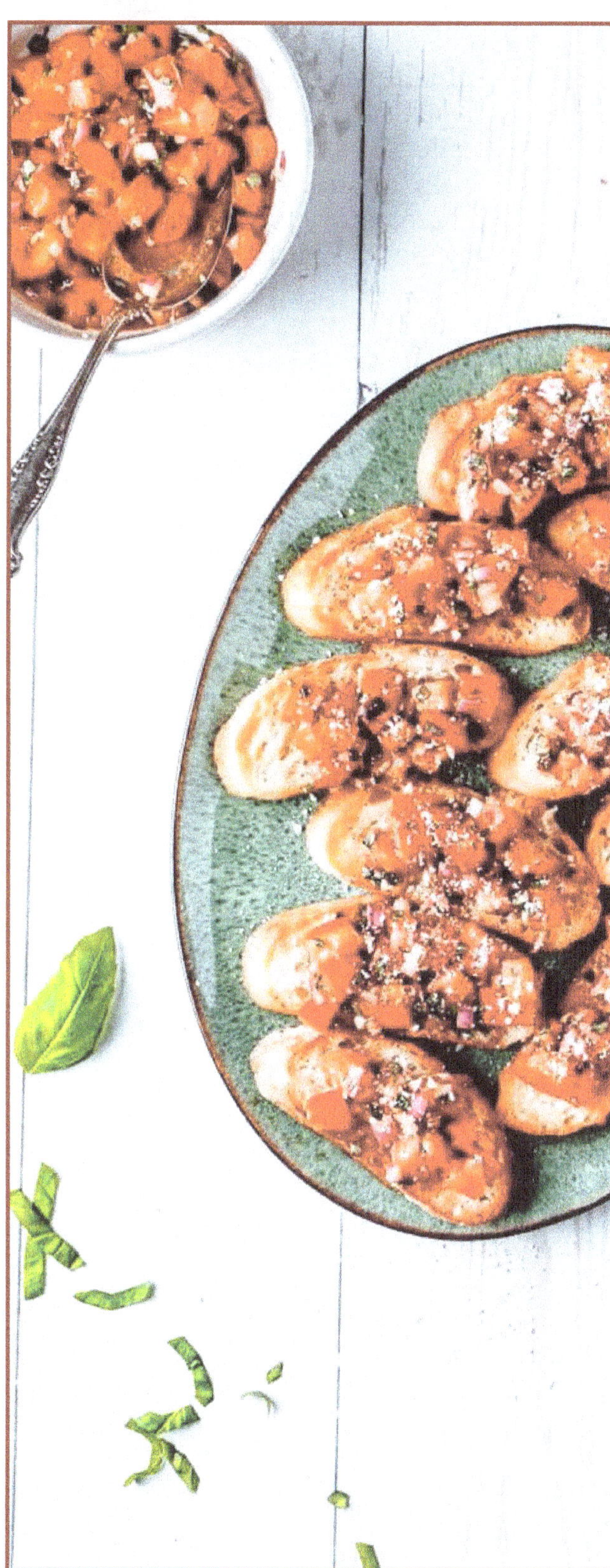

Time of Preparation: 15 minutes
Cooking Time: 5 minutes
Serving Unit: 4 servings

Ingredients:

- 4 slices of crusty bread (such as baguette or ciabatta), about 1/2 inch thick
- 2 large ripe tomatoes, diced
- 1/4 cup fresh basil leaves, chopped
- 2 cloves garlic, minced
- 2 tablespoons extra virgin olive oil
- Salt and pepper to taste

Procedures:

1. Preheat your oven broiler or grill.
2. Place the bread slices on a baking sheet and toast them under the broiler or on the grill for 1-2 minutes on each side, until golden brown and crispy.
3. In a mixing bowl, combine the diced tomatoes, chopped basil, minced garlic, and extra virgin olive oil. Season with salt and pepper to taste and toss to coat evenly.
4. Let the tomato basil mixture marinate for a few minutes to allow the flavors to meld together.
5. Once the bread slices are toasted, remove them from the oven or grill and transfer them to a serving platter.
6. Spoon the tomato basil mixture generously over each toast slice, distributing it evenly.
7. Drizzle any remaining olive oil from the mixing bowl over the bruschetta for added flavor.
8. Serve the Tomato Basil Bruschetta immediately, and enjoy!

Cooking Tips:

- Choose ripe, juicy tomatoes for the best flavor and texture in the bruschetta.

- Use fresh basil leaves for a vibrant and aromatic flavor, but you can also substitute dried basil if fresh basil is not available.
- Rub the toasted bread slices with a clove of garlic before topping them with the tomato basil mixture for an extra burst of garlic flavor.
- For added richness, you can sprinkle grated Parmesan cheese or crumbled feta cheese over the bruschetta before serving.
- Serve the bruschetta as an appetizer, snack, or light meal, either warm or at room temperature.

Nutritional Values:
- Calories: Approximately 150 kcal per serving (1 slice of bruschetta)
- Protein: Approximately 3g per serving
- Carbohydrates: Approximately 15g per serving
- Fat: Approximately 8g per serving
- Fiber: Approximately 2g per serving

Health Benefits:
- Tomatoes are rich in vitamins, minerals, and antioxidants, including vitamin C, vitamin K, and lycopene, which support immune function, bone health, and cardiovascular health, and may help reduce the risk of chronic diseases.
- Basil is an aromatic herb that's rich in vitamins A and K, as well as antioxidants, which promote eye health, bone health, and overall well-being.
- Garlic contains sulfur compounds with potential health benefits, including anti-inflammatory and antimicrobial properties, which may help boost immune function and reduce the risk of infections.
- Olive oil is a staple of the Mediterranean diet and is rich in heart-healthy monounsaturated fats and antioxidants, which may help reduce inflammation, lower cholesterol levels, and protect against heart disease and stroke.

Stuffed Bell Peppers with Quinoa

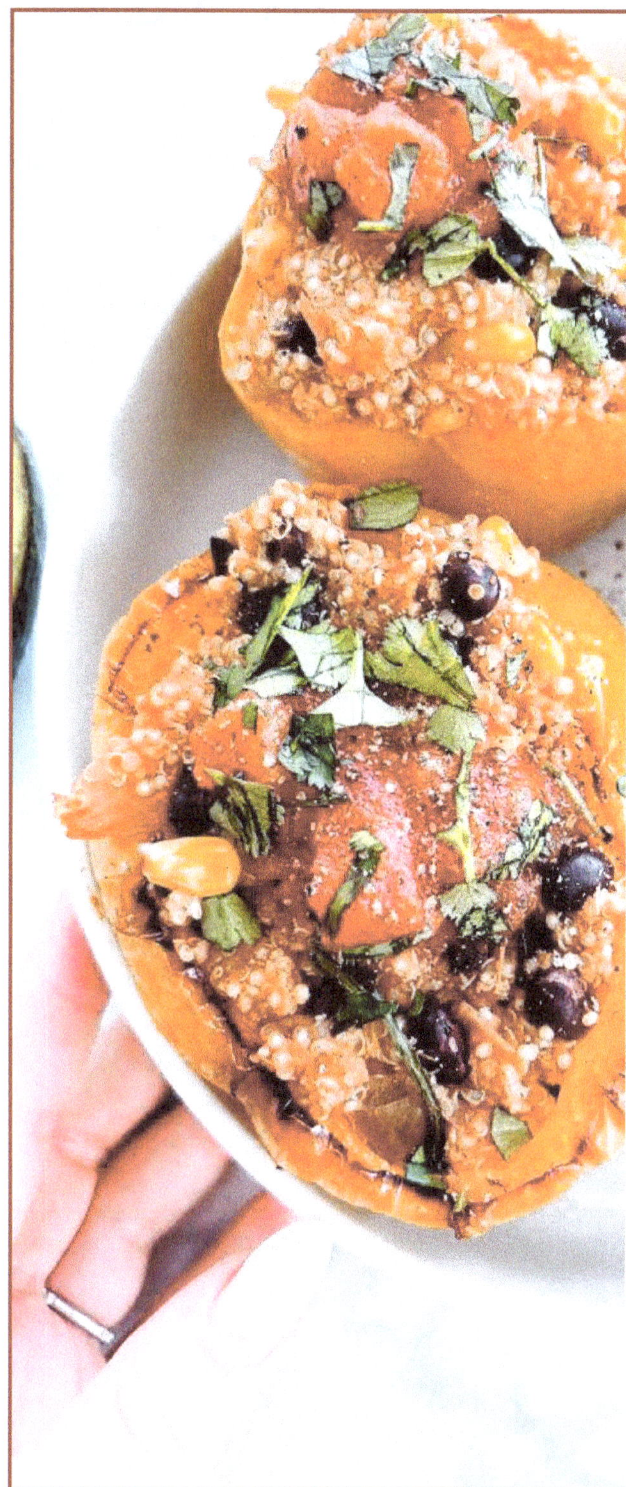

Time of Preparation: 10 minutes
Cooking Time: 20 minutes
Serving Unit: 4 servings

Ingredients:
- 4 large bell peppers, any color
- 1 cup cooked quinoa
- 1 can (14 oz) diced tomatoes, drained
- 1 cup cooked black beans
- 1/2 cup shredded cheese (such as cheddar or mozzarella)
- Optional toppings: chopped fresh cilantro, salsa, avocado, sour cream

Procedures:
1. Preheat the oven to 375°F (190°C).
2. Cut the tops off the bell peppers and remove the seeds and membranes from the inside. Rinse the peppers under cold water and pat them dry with a paper towel.
3. In a mixing bowl, combine the cooked quinoa, diced tomatoes, and cooked black beans. Stir to mix well.
4. Stuff each bell pepper with the quinoa mixture, pressing it down gently to pack it tightly.
5. Place the stuffed bell peppers upright in a baking dish or on a baking sheet lined with parchment paper.
6. Sprinkle the shredded cheese evenly over the tops of the stuffed bell peppers.
7. Cover the baking dish with aluminum foil and bake in the preheated oven for 20-25 minutes, or until the bell peppers are tender and the cheese is melted and bubbly.
8. Remove the foil during the last 5 minutes of baking to allow the cheese to brown slightly.
9. Once the stuffed bell peppers are cooked through, remove them from the

oven and let them cool for a few minutes before serving.

10. Serve the stuffed bell peppers hot, garnished with chopped fresh cilantro, salsa, avocado, and sour cream if desired.

Cooking Tips:

- Choose large bell peppers that are firm and have a flat bottom so they can stand upright in the baking dish.
- Feel free to customize the filling with your favorite ingredients, such as cooked ground meat, rice, or additional vegetables.
- Make sure to pack the quinoa mixture tightly into the bell peppers to prevent it from falling out during baking.
- For a vegan option, omit the cheese or use a dairy-free cheese alternative.
- You can prepare the quinoa mixture ahead of time and store it in the refrigerator until ready to use.

Nutritional Values:

- Calories: Approximately 250 kcal per serving (1 stuffed bell pepper)
- Protein: Approximately 10g per serving
- Carbohydrates: Approximately 30g per serving
- Fat: Approximately 10g per serving
- Fiber: Approximately 8g per serving

Health Benefits:

- Bell peppers are rich in vitamins, minerals, and antioxidants, such as vitamin C, vitamin A, and potassium, which support immune function, eye health, and heart health.
- Quinoa is a gluten-free whole grain that's high in protein, fiber, vitamins, and minerals, which support digestive health, blood sugar control, and weight management.
- Black beans are a good source of plant-based protein, fiber, vitamins, and minerals, such as folate, iron, and magnesium, which support heart health, digestion, and overall wellbeing.
- Cheese adds creaminess and flavor to the stuffed bell peppers, as well as calcium and protein, which support bone health and muscle growth.

Chapter 9: Decadent Desserts with a Healthy Twist

Chapter 9: Decadent Desserts with a Healthy Twist

Welcome to Chapter 9 where we explore the world of decadent desserts with a healthy twist. In this chapter, we prove that you can satisfy your sweet tooth without compromising your health or blood sugar levels.

Indulging in desserts doesn't have to mean sacrificing your health goals. With a few simple swaps and smart ingredient choices, you can enjoy delicious desserts that are lower in sugar, carbohydrates, and calories, while still being incredibly satisfying and indulgent.

From rich chocolate treats and creamy puddings to fruity delights and frozen delights, you'll find a variety of mouthwatering dessert recipes in this chapter that are sure to impress. Whether you're hosting a dinner party, celebrating a special occasion, or simply treating yourself to a sweet treat, these desserts are perfect for any occasion.

So go ahead, indulge your sweet cravings guilt-free with these decadent desserts with a healthy twist. You deserve it!

Flourless Chocolate Avocado Brownies

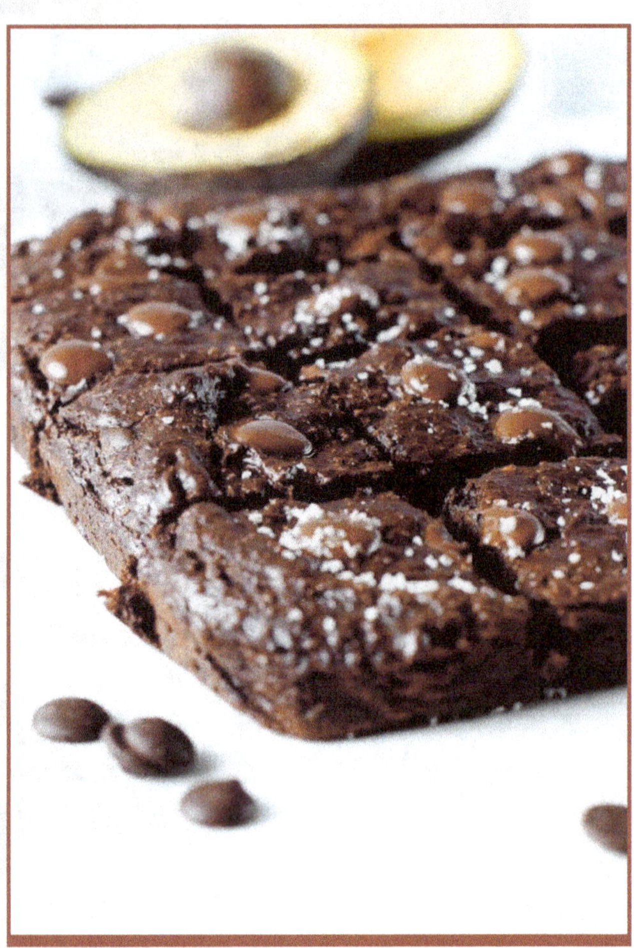

Time of Preparation: 10 minutes
Cooking Time: 20 minutes
Serving Unit: 12 brownies

Ingredients:
- 2 ripe avocados
- 1/2 cup cocoa powder
- 1/2 cup honey or maple syrup
- 2 large eggs
- 1 teaspoon vanilla extract
- Optional toppings: chopped nuts, chocolate chips, sea salt

Procedures:

1. Preheat the oven to 350°F (175°C). Grease an 8x8-inch baking dish or line it with parchment paper.
2. In a blender or food processor, combine the ripe avocados, cocoa powder, honey or maple syrup, eggs, and vanilla extract. Blend until smooth and creamy, scraping down the sides of the blender or food processor as needed.
3. Pour the brownie batter into the prepared baking dish and spread it out evenly with a spatula.
4. If desired, sprinkle the top of the brownie batter with chopped nuts, chocolate chips, or a pinch of sea salt for added flavor and texture.
5. Bake the brownies in the preheated oven for 20-25 minutes, or until the edges are set and a toothpick inserted into the center comes out with a few moist crumbs.
6. Remove the brownies from the oven and let them cool in the baking dish for at least 10 minutes before slicing and serving.
7. Once cooled, slice the brownies into squares and serve.

Cooking Tips:

- Use ripe avocados for the best texture and flavor in these brownies. They should be soft to the touch and yield slightly when pressed.
- If you prefer a sweeter brownie, you can adjust the amount of honey or maple syrup to taste.
- Be careful not to overmix the batter, as this can result in dense brownies. Blend just until all the ingredients are combined and smooth.
- Feel free to customize these brownies with your favorite toppings, such as chopped nuts, chocolate chips, or a sprinkle of sea salt.
- Store any leftovers in an airtight container in the refrigerator for up to 3 days. These brownies can also be frozen for longer storage.

Nutritional Values:

- Calories: Approximately 150 kcal per brownie
- Protein: Approximately 3g per brownie
- Carbohydrates: Approximately 15g per brownie
- Fat: Approximately 10g per brownie
- Fiber: Approximately 4g per brownie

Health Benefits:

- Avocados are a nutrient-dense fruit that's rich in healthy fats, fiber, vitamins, and minerals, such as potassium, vitamin K, and folate, which support heart health, digestion, and overall wellbeing.
- Cocoa powder is rich in antioxidants and flavonoids, which have been linked to numerous health benefits, including improved heart health, cognitive function, and mood.
- Honey or maple syrup adds natural sweetness to these brownies without the need for refined sugar, making them a healthier alternative to traditional brownies.
- Eggs provide protein, vitamins, and minerals, such as vitamin B12, vitamin D, and selenium, which support muscle growth, bone health, and immune function.

Fresh Fruit Salad with Mint Lime Dressings

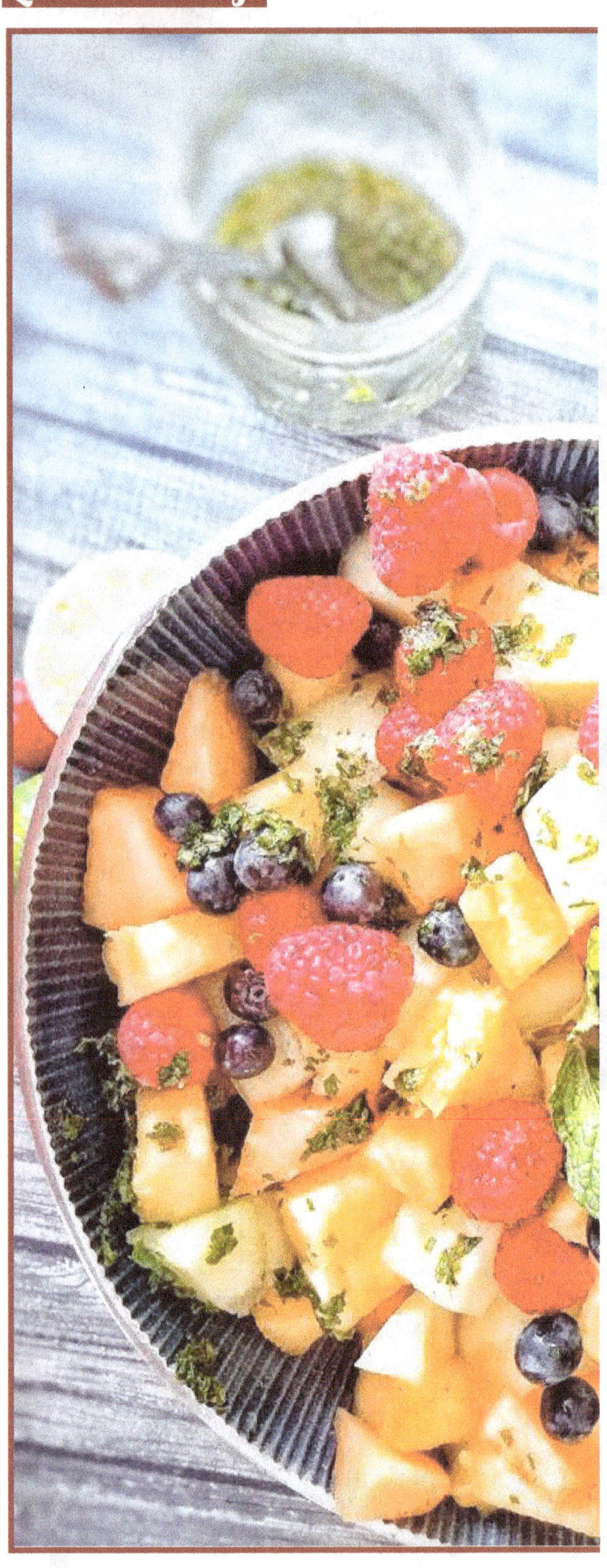

Time of Preparation: 15 minutes
Cooking Time: 0 minutes
Serving Unit: 4 servings

Ingredients:

- 2 cups mixed fresh fruit (such as strawberries, blueberries, pineapple, mango, kiwi, and grapes)
- 2 tablespoons fresh lime juice
- 1 tablespoon honey or maple syrup
- 1 tablespoon fresh mint leaves, finely chopped
- Optional garnish: fresh mint leaves, lime zest

Procedures:

1. Wash and prepare the fresh fruit as needed. Cut larger fruits like strawberries, pineapple, mango, and kiwi into bite-sized pieces. Leave smaller fruits like blueberries and grapes whole.
2. In a small bowl, whisk together the fresh lime juice, honey or maple syrup, and finely chopped mint leaves to make the dressing.
3. In a large mixing bowl, combine the mixed fresh fruit and mint lime dressing. Gently toss the fruit until it is evenly coated with the dressing.
4. Transfer the fruit salad to a serving dish or individual bowls.
5. If desired, garnish the fruit salad with additional fresh mint leaves and lime zest for added flavor and presentation.
6. Serve the fresh fruit salad immediately, or refrigerate it for up to 1 hour before serving to allow the flavors to meld.

Cooking Tips:

- Use a variety of fresh, ripe fruits for the best flavor and texture in this salad. Feel free to customize the fruit selection based on what's in season and your personal preferences.

- Adjust the amount of honey or maple syrup in the dressing to taste, depending on the sweetness of the fruit you're using.
- For extra freshness and flavor, you can add a splash of orange juice or lemon juice to the dressing.
- Serve the fruit salad chilled for a refreshing summer treat, or at room temperature for a more pronounced flavor.
- Feel free to get creative with your garnishes, such as adding toasted coconut flakes, chopped nuts, or a drizzle of balsamic glaze.

Nutritional Values:

- Calories: Approximately 80 kcal per serving
- Protein: Approximately 1g per serving
- Carbohydrates: Approximately 20g per serving
- Fat: Approximately 0g per serving
- Fiber: Approximately 3g per serving

Health Benefits:

- Fresh fruits are naturally low in calories and high in vitamins, minerals, antioxidants, and fiber, which support immune function, digestion, and overall wellbeing.
- Lime juice adds a burst of citrus flavor to the fruit salad, as well as vitamin C, antioxidants, and anti-inflammatory properties, which support immune health and skin health.
- Honey or maple syrup provides natural sweetness to the dressing without the need for refined sugar, making it a healthier option for sweetening the salad.
- Fresh mint leaves add a refreshing and aromatic flavor to the dressing, as well as digestive benefits and antimicrobial properties.

Greek Yogurt Berry Popsicles

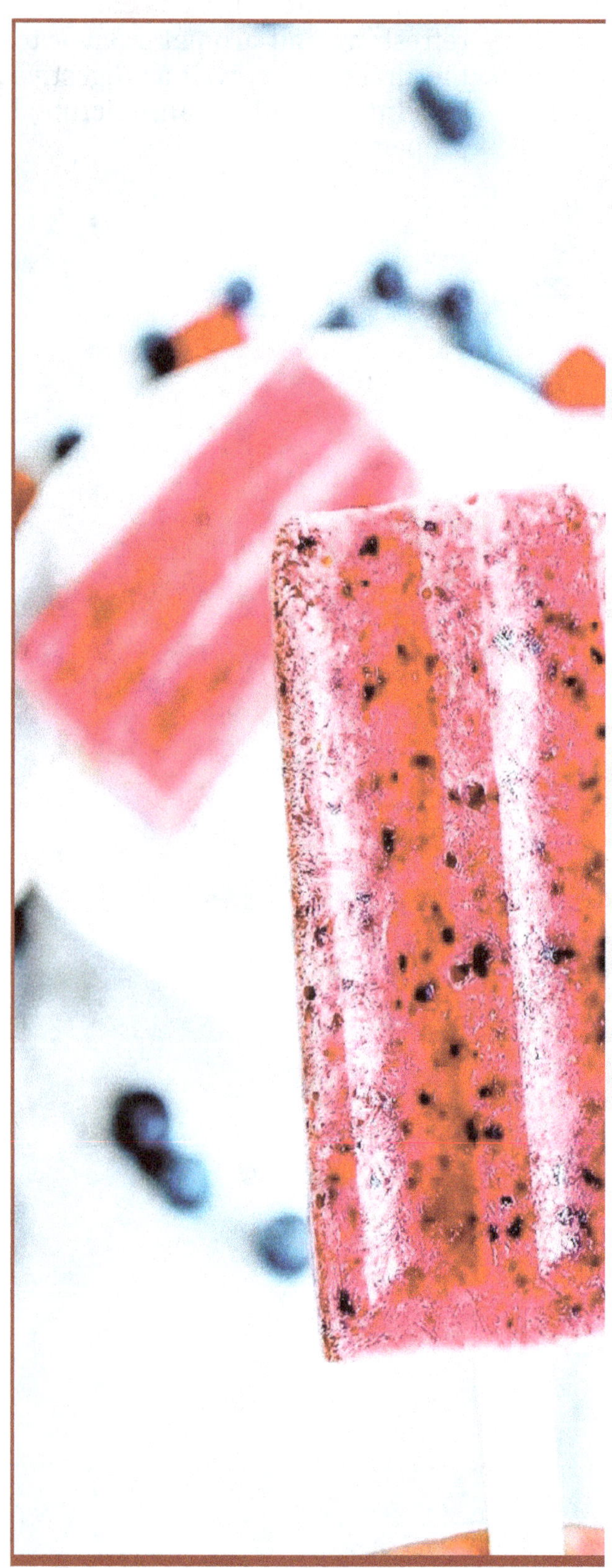

Time of Preparation: 10 minutes
Freezing Time: 4 hours
Serving Unit: Makes 6 popsicles

Ingredients:
- 1 cup Greek yogurt
- 1 cup mixed berries (such as strawberries, blueberries, raspberries)
- 2 tablespoons honey or maple syrup (optional, adjust to taste)
- 1/2 teaspoon vanilla extract (optional)
- Optional add-ins: granola, sliced almonds, shredded coconut

Procedures:
1. In a blender or food processor, combine the Greek yogurt, mixed berries, honey or maple syrup (if using), and vanilla extract (if using). Blend until smooth and well combined.
2. If desired, stir in any optional add-ins, such as granola, sliced almonds, or shredded coconut, for added texture and flavor.
3. Pour the yogurt mixture into popsicle molds, filling each mold almost to the top. Leave a little space at the top for the popsicles to expand as they freeze.
4. Insert popsicle sticks into each mold, ensuring they are centered and upright.
5. Place the popsicle molds in the freezer and freeze for at least 4 hours, or until the popsicles are completely frozen.
6. Once frozen, remove the popsicle molds from the freezer and run them under warm water for a few seconds to help release the popsicles from the molds.
7. Carefully remove the popsicles from the molds and serve immediately, or transfer them to a resealable plastic bag or container and store them in the freezer until ready to enjoy.

Cooking Tips:

- Use any combination of fresh or frozen berries that you prefer for these popsicles. Strawberries, blueberries, and raspberries are popular choices, but feel free to get creative with your selection.
- If you prefer sweeter popsicles, you can add honey or maple syrup to taste. Alternatively, you can omit the sweetener altogether if your berries are naturally sweet.
- For added flavor, you can include a splash of vanilla extract in the yogurt mixture.
- Feel free to customize these popsicles with your favorite add-ins, such as granola, sliced almonds, or shredded coconut. Simply sprinkle them into the popsicle molds before pouring in the yogurt mixture.
- To easily release the popsicles from the molds, run the molds under warm water for a few seconds before gently pulling out the popsicles.

Nutritional Values:
- Calories: Approximately 60 kcal per popsicle
- Protein: Approximately 3g per popsicle
- Carbohydrates: Approximately 8g per popsicle
- Fat: Approximately 1g per popsicle
- Fiber: Approximately 1g per popsicle

Health Benefits:
- Greek yogurt is a rich source of protein, probiotics, calcium, and vitamins, which support digestive health, bone health, and immune function.
- Berries are low in calories and high in fiber, vitamins, antioxidants, and phytochemicals, which support heart health, brain function, and overall wellbeing.
- Honey or maple syrup adds natural sweetness to the popsicles without the need for refined sugar, making them a healthier option for sweetening.
- Optional add-ins like granola, sliced almonds, or shredded coconut provide additional nutrients, such as fiber, healthy fats, and vitamins, which support energy levels and satiety.

Baked Apples with Cinnamon and Walnuts

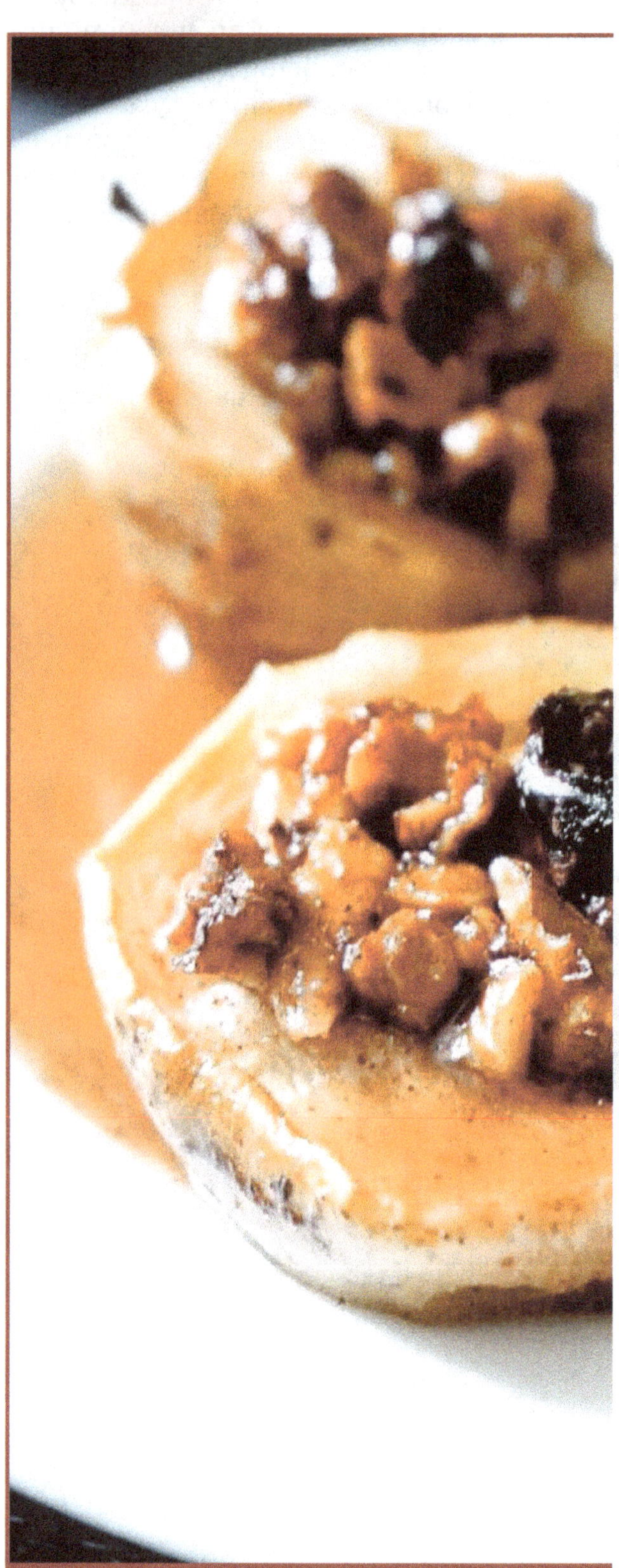

Time of Preparation: 10 minutes
Cooking Time: 20 minutes
Serving Unit: 4 servings

Ingredients:

- 4 medium-sized apples (such as Gala, Honeycrisp, or Granny Smith)
- 2 tablespoons chopped walnuts
- 1 tablespoon ground cinnamon
- 1 tablespoon honey or maple syrup (optional)
- Optional garnish: vanilla ice cream, Greek yogurt, whipped cream

Procedures:

1. Preheat the oven to 375°F (190°C). Grease a baking dish or line it with parchment paper.
2. Wash and core the apples using an apple corer or a sharp knife, leaving the bottom intact to create a well for the filling.
3. In a small bowl, mix together the chopped walnuts and ground cinnamon.
4. If desired, drizzle honey or maple syrup over the inside of each apple to add sweetness.
5. Stuff each cored apple with the cinnamon-walnut mixture, pressing it down gently to pack it tightly.
6. Place the stuffed apples upright in the prepared baking dish.
7. Bake the apples in the preheated oven for 20-25 minutes, or until they are tender and the filling is bubbly.
8. Remove the baked apples from the oven and let them cool for a few minutes before serving.
9. Serve the baked apples warm, garnished with a scoop of vanilla ice cream, a dollop of Greek yogurt, or a swirl of whipped cream if desired.

Cooking Tips:

- Choose medium-sized apples that are firm and have a sweet-tart flavor for the best results in this recipe.
- Feel free to customize the filling with your favorite nuts, such as pecans or almonds, and spices, such as nutmeg or cloves.
- If you prefer sweeter baked apples, you can drizzle honey or maple syrup over the inside of each apple before adding the filling.
- Serve the baked apples warm for a comforting dessert, or at room temperature for a lighter treat.
- Store any leftover baked apples in an airtight container in the refrigerator for up to 3 days. Reheat them in the microwave or oven before serving.

Nutritional Values:
- Calories: Approximately 120 kcal per serving (1 baked apple)
- Protein: Approximately 1g per serving
- Carbohydrates: Approximately 30g per serving
- Fat: Approximately 1g per serving
- Fiber: Approximately 5g per serving

Health Benefits:
- Apples are a good source of fiber, vitamins, and antioxidants, which support digestive health, heart health, and immune function.
- Walnuts are rich in omega-3 fatty acids, antioxidants, and vitamins, which support brain health, heart health, and inflammation control.
- Cinnamon has anti-inflammatory and antioxidant properties, which may help lower blood sugar levels, improve heart health, and reduce the risk of chronic diseases.
- Honey or maple syrup adds natural sweetness to the baked apples without the need for refined sugar, making them a healthier dessert option.

30-Day Meal Plan

Day	Breakfast	Lunch	Dinner
1	Peanut Butter Banana Smoothie	Caprese Chicken Salad	Garlic Butter Shrimp Pasta
2	Energizing Oatmeal Bowl	Tuna Salad Lettuce Wraps	Lemon Herb Chicken with Roasted Vegetables
3	Simple Greek Yogurt Parfait	Mediterranean Chickpea Salad	Cabbage and Sausage Skillet
4	Speedy Egg Muffins	Fresh Spinach and Strawberry Salad	Teriyaki Salmon with Broccoli
5	Protein-Packed Smoothie Varieties	Classic Caesar Salad with a Twist	Turkey and Sweet Potato Skillet
6	Simple Greek Yogurt Parfait	Tangy Cucumber and Tomato Salad	Sautéed Spinach and White Beans
7	Speedy Egg Muffins	Stuffed Sweet Potatoes	Veggie-Packed Quinoa Stir-Fry
8	Peanut Butter Banana Smoothie	Hearty Lentil Soup	Honey Mustard Glazed Salmon
9	Energizing Oatmeal Bowl	Creamy Tomato Basil Soup	Garlic Butter Shrimp
10	Simple Greek Yogurt Parfait	Chunky Vegetable Beef Stew	Baked Lemon Dill Tilapia
11	Speedy Egg Muffins	Chicken and Vegetable Noodle Soup	Seared Tuna Steaks with Sesame Glaze
12	Protein-Packed Smoothie Varieties	Caprese Chicken Salad	Mediterranean Style Grilled Swordfish
13	Simple Greek Yogurt Parfait	Fresh Spinach and Strawberry Salad	Herb-Roasted Chicken Thighs
14	Speedy Egg Muffins	Tuna Salad Lettuce Wraps	Honey Mustard Glazed Turkey Breast

15	Peanut Butter Banana Smoothie	Mediterranean Chickpea Salad	Lemon Garlic Chicken Skewers
16	Energizing Oatmeal Bowl	Classic Caesar Salad with a Twist	BBQ Chicken Skewers
17	Simple Greek Yogurt Parfait	Tangy Cucumber and Tomato Salad	Mushroom and Spinach Quesadillas
18	Speedy Egg Muffins	Stuffed Sweet Potatoes	Baked Cod with Herbs
19	Protein-Packed Smoothie Varieties	Caprese Chicken Salad	Stir-Fried Broccoli and Tofu
20	Simple Greek Yogurt Parfait	Fresh Spinach and Strawberry Salad	Spicy Black Bean Tacos
21	Speedy Egg Muffins	Tuna Salad Lettuce Wraps	Lentil and Vegetable Curry
22	Peanut Butter Banana	Hearty Lentil Soup	Grilled Portobello

	Smoothie		Mushroom Burgers
23	Energizing Oatmeal Bowl	Creamy Tomato Basil Soup	Tomato Basil Bruschetta
24	Simple Greek Yogurt Parfait	Chunky Vegetable Beef Stew	Stuffed Bell Peppers with Quinoa
25	Speedy Egg Muffins	Chicken and Vegetable Noodle Soup	Honey Mustard Glazed Salmon
26	Protein-Packed Smoothie Varieties	Mediterranean Chickpea Salad	Garlic Butter Shrimp
27	Simple Greek Yogurt Parfait	Fresh Spinach and Strawberry Salad	Baked Lemon Dill Tilapia
28	Speedy Egg Muffins	Tuna Salad Lettuce Wraps	Seared Tuna Steaks with Sesame Glaze

29	Peanut Butter Banana	Classic Caesar Salad	Herb-Roasted Chicken

	Smoothie	with a Twist	Thighs
30	Energizing Oatmeal Bowl	Tangy Cucumber and Tomato Salad	Lemon Garlic Chicken Skewers